Praise for Healing Naturally

Let's be honest, you can't walk three feet without tripping over a healthy lifestyle book...and since I'm always looking for a new way to deal with those weird symptoms doctors can't explain, I think I've read most of them. When I found *Healing Naturally: A Lifestyle Approach*, I assumed it would be just like the others. I knew I'd get a nugget or two, but was expecting to be rather underwhelmed. Boy, was I wrong! Rodrigues not only shares all the things we know we should be doing... but she actually tells us how to create the habits that enable us to do them! Her story is relatable and her advice is practical. I've already implemented several of her suggestions and have seen a dramatic difference in how I feel. If you want to be healthier, but you've never been able to stick to the positive habits that will help you get there, this is the book for you. Good health doesn't come in a pill, but thanks to Rodrigues, it now comes in a book.

— Sheryl Green, Mental Health Speaker and Best-selling Author of *You Had Me At No*

In her new book, Sue Rodrigues authentically shares her own personal story of moving through chronic digestive issues to illustrate that we are our *own best advocate and asset* on our own personal health journeys.

Sue's approach to building healthy habits is

invaluable. Focusing on what we do well builds confidence and trust in ourselves. Sue encourages us to find our joy while doing something good for our own long term health. Her approach also emphasizes being gentle and forgiving about our humanity. "It's good to make mistakes," because it means we are brave enough to try something at all and it is essential that we acknowledge ALL our efforts. Her approach beautifully replaces the "all or nothing approach" that can cause so many of us to sink into a sea of negativity and give up our long term health goals entirely. I know that I'd rather feel like a million bucks while championing each success and creating lifelong healthy habits.

You can easily read this book to understand how to build a holistically healthier you. A **huge bonus** is that this success building approach is applicable to many areas of our lives: for big projects that require long term goal management. It keeps the inspiration and motivation and belief in ourselves alive.

Thanks to Health Coach Sue Rodrigues' new book *Healing Naturally*, I feel inspired to revisit managing my health and well being with new hope and a new faith in myself.

— Frances Trejo-Lay Author featured in
Sanctuary (2022) & *Planting the Seed* (2023),
Women's Circle Facilitator, Reiki Practioner
and Energy Worker

Sue Rodrigues delightful and accessible book, Healing Naturally: A Lifestyle Approach, creates an path forward in focus and natural living. She gently takes her reader through her own story as well as providing easy lifestyle changes that lead to change. This beautiful book will give you solutions and focus to make the change you may not even know you need to make.

— Jessica Goldmuntz Stokes, Speaker, Educator and published Author of *Seeking Clarity in the Labyrinth, A Daughter's Journey Through Alzheimer's*, contributing Author in *Planting the Seed.*

SUE RODRIGUES

HEALING NATURALLY

a Lifestyle Approach

6 HABITS
TO SOLVE DIGESTIVE ISSUES AND THRIVE

Healing Naturally

6 Habits to Solve Digestive Issues and Thrive

Sue Rodrigues

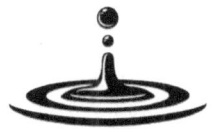

Red Thread Publishing LLC. 2024

Write to info@redthreadbooks.com if you are interested in publishing with Red Thread Publishing. Learn more about publications or foreign rights acquisitions of our catalog of books: www.redthreadbooks.com

Paperback ISBN: 979-8-218-23602-1

Ebook ISBN: 979-8-89294-010-8

Cover Design: Red Thread Designs

You understand that this book is not intended as a substitute for consultation with a licensed practitioner. Please consult with your own physician or healthcare specialist regarding the suggestions and recommendations made in this book. The use of this book implies your acceptance of this disclaimer.

Contents

Dedication

I am thrilled that I get to shout from the rooftops how fabulous my husband is! He is at his best, loving self when he is taking complete care of me. I am forever thankful for having him in my life.

John has been by my side, supporting me in both of my careers and life for the past 30 years. It is this second career, as a health coach, that I literally would not have been able to create without him being on the homefront while I changed careers after thirty years in public education to chase this dream. My health coach journey started as a hobby and grew into a side gig. I then cultivated a brand and went full-time with it. This journey took me to the most authentic place I've ever been in my life. John provided me the space and freedom to change paths and grow in a different direction. I'm sure I don't show my appreciation often enough. So here it is big time, on the decication page of my first-ever book!

John, I love you immeasurably. You have taught me that *love* is a verb. You show your love for me and our family all day, every day, without fail. You are the most consistent, stable, level-headed man I know. Our family is blessed to have you at the helm! This book is a compilation of what I've learned over the past fifteen years as I've built my health coaching career. Thank you for the space and support to learn, grow, and serve others.

Introduction

Let me tell you why I am writing this book. So many people I talk to are having digestive issues. Are you one of them? Have you had unexplained things wrong that have continued for months or years? It could be bloating, abdominal pain, acid reflux, constipation, or a ton of other ailments. Often these ailments come without a firm diagnosis. Even still, doctors offer medications that will alleviate some of these symptoms. It acts as a bandage but does not cure the issue.

Some people are OK with this disease/medication-oriented culture that exists. I am not against all medications. I'm just not in favor of long-term medications for issues that could be reduced or eliminated with healthy behaviors.

One of my pet peeves in life is the indigestion commercials where they tell you to take your antacid and continue to eat whatever you like. They show a man wrestling with a chicken wing, suggesting that this fight can be "settled" (i.e., heartburn goes away) by taking their drug.

Don't get me wrong, drugs are important and even

necessary in some instances. Due to my health-coaching experience since 2009, I understand that a lot of prescription and over-the-counter medicines are intended for lifestyle diseases that can be "cured" by cleaning up some bad habits and making better lifestyle choices if you prefer not to have the ailments or take the drugs.

Has a doctor ever given you a prescription within five minutes of hearing some of your symptoms? I get it. If, for example, a doctor gets a new patient with super-high blood pressure and something needs to be done about it immediately, a prescription may make sense. We are fortunate to have medication that will keep us from dying. However, doctors could also be giving some suggestions on how to course-correct the disease-laden paths their patients are on. Sadly, there are no nutrition courses in medical school. Neither are there classes on wellness, healthy lifestyle, or mental-health awareness unless you move on to specialize in that after you get your degree. Medical school seems to be focused on reactionary medicine; treating symptoms and fixing problems. As important as that is, wouldn't you like to see a doctor who also gets training in and focuses on creating health? Instead of just reacting to disease, they can focus on helping us thrive!

I am not writing this book to diagnose anyone or give out medical advice. Rather, I want to suggest fervently that you can work on your health to possibly reduce or eliminate your digestive issues by developing a healthier lifestyle. If it doesn't solve your digestive problems, at least you will have a healthier body! In this book, I will make the term *lifestyle* concrete and break health down into specific areas. In each area, I'll explain why it is important, what specific habits are best to start with, and how to instill them. I have been a health coach for the past fifteen years. The topics in this book are the topics I discuss every single day with my clients. I will share how to determine the habit that will be most successful for you to employ, and how to do so. In this book, I'm sharing with you everything I guide my own clients through. You may want to find a health coach of your own to assist you in building your new habits. I will write more about accountability further along in the book, and, of course, I include a coach as an excellent option. There are other options we'll take a look at, too.

I beg the question, how can we take charge of our health?

Yes, see your doctors. Good healthcare providers should be on your health team. It is us, the patients, who are the head coaches of our healthcare teams. The medical staff are the quarterbacks. We need to be our advocates and **lead** the team. The physicians have been trained. They know way more than we do in each of their specialized areas. No doubt about that. However, we are individuals. Doctors may see trends because they are in the trenches all day. They see patterns. They typically assume that our case is going to be the same as most others. It seems to me that prescribing drugs is their go-to, while they are trying to figure out your disease or ailment. Hopefully, they run a myriad of tests to either rule out or find the cause of your symptoms. Their routine way of dealing with medical issues seems to have us at their mercy. Again, I want to reiterate that quality providers are essential. They are not bad at their jobs for prescribing meds. I simply want to encourage you to do your research as well. Only you know all your specific symptoms. Google them to see what could be wrong with you, then share your information with your doctor. The doctor can run certain tests to confirm or deny what you've found and go from there. You will be getting to know your body better and you'll be giving the doctor a running start. Your health is a team effort with **you** at the helm.

Have you had many medications prescribed to you without a firm diagnosis? It is annoying and frustrating to live with continual, unexplained pain. It compounds the frustrations of having to take daily prescription drugs based on a hunch of what may be wrong. Have you been given an over-the-counter (OTC) or prescription drug even though the doctor didn't have a firm diagnosis for you? "Acid reflux" is one of those diagnoses when there are digestive upsets with no real hardcore certainty. What is prescribed? You name it: Omeprozole, Famitid, and a myriad of other OTC digestive drugs. If the drug gives you relief, I'm all for it. I don't like to be in pain or be in discomfort either. I just wish more attention would also be given to figure out the **cause** of the pain or discomfort. Imagine the cause being addressed and fixed! There would be less of a need for lifetime medicines. Instead of simply reacting to the ailments and being put on medications for a lifetime, root causes and course corrections could be implemented.

This is why it's important to create habits that focus on what you want to create in your life, not what you want to run away from. Do you know what I mean by that? Instead of taking lifelong meds for high cholesterol, how about learning how to eat in such a way as to lower your (bad) cholesterol numbers? I get it: some people will need the drugs no matter what. However, the statistics seem to prove that good nutrition and healthy lifestyle habits can work wonders in reducing cholesterol as well as many other diseases and illnesses for the majority. It makes sense, right? Many times, diabetes is developed in individuals who eat a lot of sugar, which—besides being inflammatory throughout the body—can throw off your insulin and glucose levels creating the illness. This isn't true 100% of the time, but enough times to recognize that behaviors need to change to self-correct and create better health. This is the ultimate reason for the book. My digestive issues, as you'll read about later, spawned the idea of helping people with digestive issues. I'm hoping this book helps all people with or without digestive issues. This is for anyone who needs direction and motivation in striving for their best health.

I will begin this book with my story about my unsolved digestive issue during the past ten years. See what parts you can relate to. Sometimes when you read someone else's journey, it can help to clarify your own. Perhaps it can validate your journey and your emotions. I hope you find encouragement in my story. I had ten years of undiagnosed digestive issues. Ten years. My goodness. I am a health coach and I couldn't figure it out. Good health is my passion and my expertise. Yet, I couldn't figure out what was wrong with me, and neither could any doctors. I was frustrated and exhausted, to say the least. I was finally diagnosed in 2022 when I made solving this pain-inducing health mystery of mine a major goal for the year. It's quite a story. If you'd rather skip that part and go right to part where I help you create and install healthy habits, be my guest. This is your journey.

In the second part of the book, I will help you with all of this. I will give you many areas in which you can work, one at a time, focusing on the areas you need most. We will explore the benefits and how you can create success by embracing these habits. Habit implementation is the biggest roadblock most people face. I won't necessarily be telling you anything new. Let's face it, we all know what to do. Rather, I will be guiding you on how to get healthy in a baby-step approach so that change can become sustainable. You do not have to suffer anymore. Who's up for that? Buckle up. Here we go!

Part 1
My Story

I share my story with you in the hopes that you may see parts of your story in mine. I hope it validates your journey and helps to guide you on the path to getting yourself healed. As you read, you'll see that sometimes one thing you read, or one comment a person makes, can be enough to change your course of action and lead to a diagnosis and finally a cure. If you relate to my story, maybe they'll be some thing trajectory changing in it for you.

Chapter 1
The Beginning

My annoyance of our culture turning to a medication instead of taking preventive measures to bypass the need for medications, actually turned into a philosophy, a career, and a lifestyle. It started in 2008 when I was told by my primary care physician, after a review of my blood work, that I was going to have to go on medication to lower my cholesterol. I said I did not want to do that, so she said she would give me two months to see if I could turn it around. She did not give me a game plan. She offered me no alternatives to the medications; rather, she sent me off to figure things out on my own. I happened to call my brother to complain about my predicament. He suggested that I try the weight-loss program he was offering his patients in his chiropractic practice. Well, I was offended because I thought he was calling me fat. You can't blame me for that, right? He knew, though, that high cholesterol often has a lot to do with what we eat, and learning to eat more healthfully would certainly help. I was willing to try anything that didn't involve drugs. Has this happened to you? Have you been prescribed drugs by your physician as the only remedy to your digestive ailment? It seems to be the norm. We follow doctors' orders because they are trained professionals. It's understandable.

Chapter 2
Radical Responsibility

My siblings and I grew up with a mother whose weight skyrocketed post-pregnancy. During her journey toward obesity, I was taught at an early age that eating was fun. Eating was entertainment. Eating was a way to escape reality for a while. My goodness, there were some Sunday nights when we all got as much ice cream as we wanted for dinner. When my friends would come over for sleepovers my mom bought big brown grocery bags filled with candy for our entertainment. I even remember when we were little our babysitters would give us candy to stay in our rooms all night. Can you imagine that? Of course, we figured out a way to get all the candy and sneak into each other's rooms anyway. But I digress. The point is, when asked if I was a healthy eater, I always said "yes." My three meals each day were healthy. I did not count the pint of Ben and Jerry's ice cream while I was watching American Idol three days a week as part of my "food" intake; it was part of my "entertainment." What a surprise that my cholesterol was high. Not! *Of course* my cholesterol was high. I didn't need medication. I needed to bring my ice-cream consumption to a halt. Not realizing that at the time and feeling desperate to try anything, I tried the weight-loss program my brother told me about. After eight weeks I went back to the doctor's office. She was amazed by my progress. I had lost eighteen pounds, which I didn't know I needed to lose. And I lowered my overall cholesterol by a whopping fifty points. She gave me praise and told me to keep up the great work, and that I didn't need to take any medications.

It was at this point that I had two major, trajectory-changing epiphanies. One was that I could be delusional. By that I mean, I can unknowingly bury my head in the sand and believe things that aren't true to stay comfortable. I didn't even think I had any weight to lose when I was getting healthy. I was solely going on this weight-loss program to lower my cholesterol. Sure, my clothes were getting tight but....get ready for this...I thought my dryer wasn't working and it was shrinking my clothes. Talk about not taking responsibility. Oh my goodness! Talk about burying your head in the sand. Do you do the same thing? You know...make excuses for why things are the way they are that does not include you having anything to do with it? This was about to change as I was about to go down a path of radical responsibility. In other words, I was about to take ownership of all my life's circumstances, even my high cholesterol!

Secondly, I learned to connect the dots. For example, eating at night, those calories didn't count, right? I thought if people didn't see me eat, it didn't count. If I am eating the leftover crust from my daughter's grilled cheese, that doesn't count as food intake, right? I know this sounds crazy. Do you remember the low-fat craze in the 80s? Well, half of America gained weight. Why? They thought delusionally, too. They thought that if a snack is low in fat, it must be low in calories and therefore okay to eat a whole box of cookies. Another example of taking responsibility for your outcomes is in the workplace. Everything you do at a job has a consequence, right? You do well, you get a raise. You do poorly and you could be fired. The same with students in the classroom. If they work hard and study, they get good grades. If they are absent a lot or don't do their work, their grades will be below par. It is easy to see that. I'm not sure why we fail to connect the dots with our health and our daily habits. Perhaps many people are just like I was. I did not connect the dots. I remember going to happy hours on Fridays with my teacher friends and having fun. When I got healthy and changed my habits, I saw happy hour as a place to drink alcohol (which I knew I didn't want to do anymore), eating fried foods (which I wasn't eating anymore), and complaining about other teachers, students, parents and administrators (which I didn't want to partake in anymore). It was a negative environment and I hadn't even recognized that because I was immersed in the culture. I thought that happy hour was the reward at the end of the week. Again I used all these unhealthy habits as something that was entertaining and had nothing to do with my health when, in fact, it was bringing me down in body, mind, and spirit. I would come home tired after a Friday evening happy hour, go to sleep early, and wake up late Saturday morning. Recuperating from the alcohol and food was taking time out of my family life. How could I have not realized all this before?

Well, it can take just one incident—like my doctor telling me I have to go on meds. I was so vehemently against that idea that it began to change the trajectory of my whole life! I stopped going to happy hours and life improved immediately.

Literally. With something as simple as having a full evening with my family and having energy on Saturday mornings. And this was just the beginning of what has come to be my perpetual health journey. And by perpetual, I don't mean learning the same things over and over again. I mean continually striving for more. It's like when you climb a mountain and you're so happy that you reached the top. This, however, gives you a vantage point and you can see another peak. Now you can get back on the path to strive for more. You have already **become** more. Now you can see more for yourself. It puts us in lifelong-learner mode, which is a wonderful place to be. You can continually celebrate progress and personal wins while also setting new goals. This develops a sense of pride by reaching and attaining many accomplishments along the way, and this never ceases. Can't we all use a bit more self-love and confidence? Sure we can. Being true to your word and doing something you promised yourself you would do is the way to build up your self-esteem. Becoming more capable is the reward we get along the way.

To be honest, I do not make healthy decisions 100% of the time. Who does? Sometimes I go to happy hour, sometimes I eat ice cream, sometimes I eat junk food. What I have learned is that it is what you do **most** of the time that matters. One cheeseburger will not make you fat. One salad will not make you healthy. In an attempt to live life and not be too extreme, this is the philosophy that guides me: make good choices most of the time. With a newfound sense of health and self-awareness, I went along my merry way for several years taking radical responsibility for my choices. I have come to realize that everything I do has a cause and an effect. If I am not satisfied with where my body and health are, I need to look at the actions that may have brought me there. If we can all connect the dots, and not bury our heads in the sand, perhaps we can get to the core of our digestive issues faster. Of course, solving digestive issues isn't as clear-cut as lowering cholesterol. Lowering cholesterol can be done because we get a diagnosis telling us that our cholesterol is high. Chances are if you're reading this book, you have digestive issues of an unknown origin. Your challenge right now is to figure out what it is so you can get a diagnosis and take the necessary action steps to alleviate your symptoms. I will highlight the steps I took to get my diagnosis in the hopes that something along my path will spark an idea for you to follow. If I can get a diagnosis, I know it is possible for you, too. My story may have a step or a direction to get you on the road to recovery sooner than later. Let's get after it for you, too.

Chapter 3
First Incident

About four years after lowering my cholesterol and losing eighteen pounds, I had another trajectory-changing incident.

I was at a school picnic on a staff-development day. There were just teachers and staff in the building. At the picnic, we had the usual food: hamburgers, hot dogs, potato chips, potato salad, and cookies. Not the usual food for me, but I imbibed with everyone else. After socializing a bit we all met in different classrooms with the other teachers in our grade levels to accomplish our assigned tasks.

A few minutes in, I started to feel strange. I started getting clammy and sweaty. I felt a tightness in my chest that was scary because it was painful and I felt like I couldn't breathe. One gal was rubbing my shoulders to calm me down. I turned white and they all got scared. Unbeknownst to me, they called the paramedics who arrived soon after this "attack" started. They took my vitals, put me in an ambulance, and got me to the ER of the local hospital as fast as they could. The worry was that I was having a heart attack. They gave me every kind of test imaginable and found nothing. It was not my heart, they could attest to that. As I processed what had happened to me, I was at a loss. The hospital pronounced me healthy. I just figured that the high-fat burgers and all the fat-laden food from the school picnic caused a reaction and I went back to my normal, healthy ways. I had a follow-up visit with a doctor in my HMO and they also found nothing wrong.

Chapter 4
Next Episode

The next episode didn't happen for at least seven months. When it happened again, I kind of panicked. It's such a scary situation. I was in a restaurant eating a low-fat meal. As my friend was talking to me, I started to feel funny. I felt a discomfort in my chest. All of a sudden my bra was too tight. It felt like I couldn't breathe well. I started sweating. I told my friend I had to leave because I had to get to the car to take my bra off. She was worried, and told me to go.

When I got to the car, I immediately unlatched my bra and undid my pants button. I was now in full sweat clutching my chest with a pressure-like kind of pain. I didn't know whether to ride it out and sit in the car until it was over or drive to a drug store and get some acid blockers. I knew it wasn't my heart even though the pain felt like it was right at the sternum. I guess I figured that it may be acid reflux although it didn't feel like anything was coming up from the stomach. The pain felt like it was radiating from my chest. I waited a few minutes and because nothing was improving, I drove to the nearest drug store and got an acid blocker. I took it immediately. I recovered within minutes. So I figured that the acid blocker worked.

When I told my pharmacist friend that the acid blocker worked almost immediately, she said that the medicine did not work that fast. She figured I was most likely having a panic attack. This made no sense to me because I am a low-key and relaxed person. I don't have much stress in my life. But I started wondering if I had some underlying issues that I wasn't addressing.

I couldn't figure out any underlying causes of these attacks. I was calling them heart attacks because I imagined that this was what a heart attack would feel like. I **knew** it wasn't my heart because of the testing I had done. But I did clutch my chest when I had the attacks. They were happening more often. I turned to Tums and acid blockers. I never knew when it was going to happen, but I knew I needed them close by for quick relief. I was starting to get the attacks so frequently that I could tell when they were going to come on. I'd start to feel uncomfortable, like I ate too much. Then a pain in the back of my shoulder blade, the sweating came next, and soon a full feeling of chest constriction. No position was comfortable. Pain was in the form of feeling like I couldn't take a breath because something was just so tight in the chest area. Sometimes nausea would come, but not always. They would last about twenty to thirty minutes and they were followed by sheer exhaustion. I knew that my body was trying to handle these attacks as best it could, but they took a toll on me. I was popping Tums and other acid blockers left and right. I had some in the car, on my nightstand by my bed, in the bathroom, and the living room. Until one day, I said, "this isn't right. I can't live like this with this kind of pain and discomfort." The doctors said nothing was wrong. I had to figure it out on my own. I noticed that spicy foods weren't feeling or tasting good anymore. I felt bloated and full after I ate them. Certainly, it appeared to me that my digestion was changing. Foods and drinks that I enjoyed were no longer tasting or feeling good. The problem seemed to be growing. Could this be just an aging process? I wondered if maybe I need to eat less, or avoid spicy food and/or meat. I was at a loss, but knew I had to figure something out.

Chapter 5
My Google Education

With no clear idea of what was going on in my body, I started my education on digestive issues. I had to figure it out myself. Enter "University of Google." My mom was the queen of self-diagnosis via the internet—mostly on WedMD. I took her legacy and extended it to include all of the internet! I am guessing that you have done this a few times yourself. Don't we all?

My first hunch was that I had low digestive enzymes. I started piecing things together with this hypothesis. I read that as you get older, your digestive enzymes can decrease and foods become harder to digest. This felt like it could be the cause of my ailments. I began researching what to do with low stomach acid. The big answer seemed to be to eat an alkaline-based diet. So I read up on all the things and decided to drink warm, salted, lemon water each morning and eat a vegan diet. (Believe it or not, lemon juice is acidic on its own, but when digested it becomes alkaline in the body.) I learned that meat and dairy are acidic and make the body work very hard to digest them. I started to watch some of the vegan documentaries to fuel my desire to eat in this new way, and it worked. I ate separately from my family for about seven months. I also realized I hadn't had an attack in all that time, so I felt I had found the answer to my problem by eating an alkaline diet.

It was seven months filled with learning a new lifestyle. I became friends with lots of vegans in the Las Vegas community. I started cooking my food. I loved it. It was a creative time with a steep learning curve into a whole new lifestyle. The only tiny problem was that I was gaining weight. Why, you ask? Well, I became delusional again. I wasn't even eating a lot of vegetables. I had Cinnaholic cinnamon rolls, frozen fake crab cakes, vegan pizza, and lots of ice cream... non-dairy, but filled with calories and fat. I wasn't monitoring the quantity or quality of my food. I just made sure it was low acid. Then I got another attack, so I knew I had to revamp things. I decided to redefine my veganism to incorporate way more fruits, veggies, legumes, and grains. I stopped eating the fake meats, and high-sugar snacks and went to a truly whole-foods, plant-based (WFPB) style of eating. Meaning sugar would come from food, not from an added ingredient. Trust me, I wasn't an absolutist, but about 90% of my food choices were WFPB. As a result, I lost the seven pounds I gained in the first seven months I went vegan. I was back to being pain-free with no attacks. I thought I had it all figured out again until I got my next attack about five months later. I tried to figure out what I did wrong. Did I drink coffee? Have something minty? Too much chocolate? Something carbonated? All things that were known to instigate acid reflux, which was still on the table as a possibility of being my issue. It was something digestive, I was sure of that. But that's all I knew for sure.

I decided to start documenting my episodes. I wanted to see if I could draw any connections to what I weighed, how much I ate, what I ate, and who I was with. Perhaps with documentation, I could see some sort of patterns developing. Any time I had an attack, I figured whatever I had just done was causing it. And I'd aim not to do that again.

No one could tell me what was wrong. These scary, painful, sweaty attacks were still unexplained. I was alone in my diagnosis because traditional medicine wasn't helping to solve the mystery. On the positive side of it, however, was how much I learned about health, wellness, and nutrition. I learned that I am my number-one line of defense. In essence, it was my medical experiment. I chose to hone my daily rituals, which is where all the magic lies. I will get into it in depth in the second part of this book so you can benefit from all that I learned.

Pain is not normal. Usually, we just take a drug to take the pain away. Pain is an indicator that something is not right. We need to pay attention to it and learn from it—just like with a car. When the engine light comes on in our car, we don't cut the wire that shows us the warning light; we take it in for diagnosis and repair. Having had no luck with the medical delivery system, I tried what I could to diagnose myself to no avail. I'd go seven or eight months sometimes without an attack and I thought I was onto something. But disappointingly, the attacks would strike again and I was back to playing detective and doctor all rolled into one. It took ten years before I went back to try the medical route again because what I was doing was not solving my digestive issues. True, the attacks were fewer and further apart, but they were still a heavy part of my mind's landscape about being careful about everything I ingested. It was a constant worry. I always wondered, would I be out in public when it happened again? I would be so careful ordering food in a restaurant while being out with others. I didn't want to have an attack out with friends. Of course, it happened several times with friends over the ten years.

Chapter 6
2022 Goal and Action Steps

By the end of 2021, I had two of my lifelong friends pass away from cancer. While it was devastatingly sad, I was also realizing that time on this planet is just way too short. I was turning 60, which was a very big deal for me. (And on top of that we were having a bathroom renovated which, of course, brought on another host of stressors.) I was emotionally raw. I was allowing my emotions to flow when they needed to and taking all the time I needed to process and feel all the feelings. With my lifestyle, I was able to just stop, sit, and cry if I needed to. Interestingly, sadness became a friend. It was painful and at the same time comforting, if that makes sense. At the same time, I knew I wasn't living my best physical health. One thing I knew for sure from being a health coach for the past fifteen years, is that health is a series of small habits strung together to create magic. It's not just diet and exercise. I had that down. My mindset was very positive and grounded. I was good in the mental gym. I meditated, journaled, and remained grateful. Still, there was something I needed more to crack the case of my digestive mystery.

I made my goal for 2022 to solve my digestive issue once and for all. It was my number-one task for the year. That would be the *one* habit I would incorporate and make a top priority to achieve. I was giving myself the whole year to accomplish it.

In the meantime, one of my friends of more than thirty years, Myriam, told me about this energy healer in Vegas. She has a good friend who has seen him for years. He is very sought-after and it's hard to get an appointment to see him. I figured what the heck, let me try to get an appointment and see what happens. If it's only for entertainment purposes it would still be fun to get a reading and have the possibility of healing. My energy-healing friend, Debra, suggested that I go in prepared with several questions in different areas of my life to ask questions in the hopes of releasing anything that wasn't serving me.

I got my appointment in November of 2021. I met the healer. I was a little nervous because I had no idea what to expect. After just a few minutes, I knew this guy was amazing. He "cut chords" to things I was attached to for my whole life. I was having shoulder pain. After eliminating physical causes for it, he told me that it was a sign of grieving or an emotionally broken heart. This, of course, made total sense to me because I was broken hearted after losing my two best, oldest, closest friends in the whole world within six months of each other. So after that, everything he said continued to be spot-on and were real aha moments for me. I could write a whole book just about that one experience!! But the biggest shock of what he told me, which I blew off and disagreed with, was that he suggested I take a look at my gallbladder because he thought "something might be up with it." I connected with everything else he told me except that! So I just left it there... for the time being.

Chapter 7
Finding a Thorough Doctor

I asked one of my very good friends, Dawn, who is a model of excellence with meticulous standards, who her doctor was. She had lots of issues with her health over the years and I remember her always saying how thorough her doctor was and how much time she gave her patients. So I got an appointment for the start of 2022.

Fresh and ready to get right on my goal of 2022, I had my first appointment with the nurse practitioner. He spent about ninety minutes with me. He asked questions about every aspect of my health history. I told him my main reason for coming in was to solve this digestive issue I was having that I thought might be acid reflux. He started with all the labs, and lots of testing to see what was happening on the inside of my body. It was the most thorough examination I have ever had. Can you imagine a primary-care provider taking that much time? He did and he was very thorough about every part of my health. I was thankful he took so much time with me and felt good that I had a solid start in the direction of my 2022 health goal.

In the following weeks, data was being collected, and I scheduled a follow-up to go over everything. I got the blood results before I had my follow-up. My mom, when she was alive, was very interested in lab results, so I knew my way around reading these reports. As I was looking happily over my great results, I noticed that my amylase was low. I had no idea what that was so I went back to my old faithful, University of Google, and began researching. I found out that amylase is a digestive enzyme. Aha! My original hypothesis was true. I had figured that I had low digestive enzymes based on researching my symptoms. I was beginning to think that this was another one of those aging things (you know, like getting stiff if you sit too long, or needing bifocals...and the list goes on. Oy.) I didn't stop my research there.

Amylase is an enzyme found in the pancreas. So I looked up reasons why amylase could be low. It pointed to the pancreas, and specifically, pancreatitis. As I looked further into that illness, a lot of the symptoms did not match what I was experiencing. So I kept looking. I canceled out pancreatic cancer because I had none of those symptoms either. One possible cause of pancreatitis is gallstones. And then it dawned on me; the energy healer suggested I check out my gallbladder a couple of months earlier. With this realization, I started looking up gallbladder issues. I came across the symptoms of gallstones. Every. Single. Symptom. Was one I had. I knew the attacks were coming when I got an increasing pain in my shoulder blade on my right side. Even that was listed! The sweatiness, vomiting, abdominal pain, burping, and feeling bloated. They were all listed there in black and white.

I felt like I finally had my answer. No more wondering what I was doing wrong, or if it was all in my mind, or worrying if it was my heart. I was excited to go back to my doctor. I realized that my Google search was not 100% certain, but I was happy to be able to share my findings at my upcoming appointment.

As I had predicted, my doctor respected my hunch and scheduled a sonogram. Within a couple of weeks, I had the sonogram and reviewed the results with my doctor. He said that there was a "mass" in my gallbladder that was about 2 ½ inches big. He didn't want to call it a gallstone because it was so unusually large. I wasn't worried because I knew that it was a gallstone. Because the doctor could not say definitively, I needed to get a CAT scan next. This took place in early March.

Getting the CAT scan was a little scary for me, but I was thrilled to be getting a (literal) clearer picture of my gallbladder. Surely this will be definitive. Then we can get on with what treatment options I had available to me. In the meantime I was going to my standard, healing procedures: a plant-based diet; yoga (for gallbladder health); breathing; and meditation to get my mind, my spirit, and my digestive system as calm as I could.

You're not going to believe it, but the sonogram was "inconclusive." The shape and size of this mass were not typical for a gallstone. My doctor felt he did all that he could do to help diagnose it and without being able to define exactly what it was, and he referred me to a surgeon he held in high regard. My mind was reeling because I know what happens when you go to a surgeon; they recommend surgery, of course. Nevertheless, I made the appointment. While I was waiting for the appointment, I started researching the doctor's credentials and possible treatments for gallstones. I wasn't going to do any of the treatments before I met with the surgeon on the outside chance that the "mass" was not a gallstone.

I had my husband, John, come with me so we would have two pairs of ears to hear what the surgeon had to say, and two minds to think of questions for him. We brought him all the results of the tests I had taken. I thought maybe with his expertise he would be able to interpret the results better than my doctor. I was wrong. He said that he has been removing gallstones and taking out gallbladders for over thirty years and he has never seen a gallstone this shape and this big. Regardless of what it was, the gallbladder needed to be taken out. He said there was no way to take out a mass that big. The word *mass* was starting to take its toll on me emotionally and I asked him if he thought it was cancer. Because the mass was not attached to the wall of the gallbladder, he was confident that it was not cancer. Still, he strongly suggested removal. On a side note, he thought that even with removing the gallbladder, there was only a 10% chance that my attacks would be cured. He thought that due to my descriptions and where the pain was coming from, it was possible that my issues were esophageal. Immediately I knew this could not be right, but he scheduled another exam with dye to see how my esophagus was working when I swallowed liquid. He also scheduled an endoscopy to be performed at the same time as my gallbladder removal surgery. That was the first action step. If he saw esophageal issues, we would tackle that next.

By the end of April, I was feeling well taken care of. I felt that there was a thorough investigation of what was going on inside of me. Some of the tests were scary and some hurt a little. Overall, I thought it was cool that our medical-delivery system could go inside and **see** how my body parts were functioning. I was feeling grateful. Just four months into my yearly goal I was getting close to solving my ten-year medical mystery.

Chapter 8
Next Was Surgery

I was heavily involved with my insurance agent (Heather, the best in all the land), and she was coaching me on the financial end of the surgery. That in and of itself could be yet another whole book. Suffice it to say, the surgery needed to be paid in full before the surgery. There were lots more bills to be paid for: x-rays, exams, lab work, and the list goes on. But I had to pay for the actual surgery and prepay the surgeon. I did all this the Friday before the surgery along with last-minute chest x-rays and general exams making sure I was still fit for surgery. I was.

As I waited, I was both nervous and excited. Nervous because I was having surgery and a worried mind can think of a million things that could go wrong. I was excited, too, because this may be the answer to all my prayers. Either the gall bladder removal will be a success and end all my unexplained digestive issues, or perhaps the endoscopy would identify some issue that escaped other tests and my extended research.

I did all the meditation I could. I focused on my desired outcomes. I kept positive, and finally the time came to go to the hospital.

Chapter 9
Signs from the Universe

Do you ever notice signs from the Universe? Ya know, like when you are thinking of someone and they mysteriously call you out of the blue, or you happen to run into someone you wanted to see. Or maybe you asked for a sign and a butterfly passes by as you're asking for a sign... that's what I'm talking about. You can choose to believe that all of those things are coincidences. I believe there are no coincidences. I believe that when these serendipitous events happen, it's a nod from the Universe that you are in alignment with your highest self, validating where you are and what you're doing.

The first sign was that the nurse taking care of me was named Edna, which happened to be my grandmother's name. I figured it meant she was watching over me and my mom was probably with her, too. The nurse took me to an area to get hooked up to monitors and put in IVs, which was room 24. I was born on the 24th. I took that as a good sign, too.

My worries were decreasing as I was feeling more and more confident that this was exactly where I needed to be.

Then what happened next? I was wheeled to operation room #7! Everyone knows that seven is a lucky number. I made it! I knew all my worries would be over as soon as I got to the OR. All I had to do was get the anesthesia... and wait to wake up in the recovery room.

Part 2
My Healing

I was already starting to realize that healing was about to come to me in many shapes, forms, and sizes. Physical healing, of course, but also, spiritually, and emotionally. In this part of the book, I'll share both.

Chapter 10
Physical Healing

It all began in that recovery room. The nurse was trying to wake me up and get me going. As I opened my eyes, I knew I made it. Phew! Ok. A giant moment of gratitude. Then, I briefly got annoyed with this nurse pushing me to get up. Get up? Really? I just came out of surgery. But, I understood. They have to clear beds and make way for the next wave of patients. In an attempt to bring me back to anesthesia-free consciousness, she started to tell me how she had her gallbladder out (which, by the way, so many people had been telling me since I found out I was having the surgery) and warned me about having to run to the restroom with diarrhea after eating a bacon cheeseburger. She claimed that when people don't have a gallbladder they have difficulty metabolizing fats. My surgeon, however, said I would be able to eat normally after I recover from the surgery once I healed, so I was a little perplexed and concerned about her comment. Once I was off my post-op liquid-based recovery diet, I was determined to slowly try **all** the food and drink I had avoided for years that were high in fat, spicy, caffeinated, and contained alcohol and prove this nurse wrong.

So home I went, excited to fully embrace the following two weeks of healing. The first day or so was managing pain. I was fine if I didn't move, which I tried not to do most of the day. John took the best care of me and my every little need, so I didn't have to do much. Once the muscle relaxer kicked in, I was able to get up and go to the bathroom on my own. On day two, I stopped taking the muscle relaxer and went to Motrin, so that was a major improvement. The strong drugs made me very groggy, and I didn't like that. I was only feeling pain when I got up from a lying or sitting position. On day three, I did a little bit of business, had a Zoom meeting, and answered some texts.

Some people say that recovery is just a few days, but I was listening very carefully to my body and did not try to do too much. I remember the first time I drove about a week after surgery—yowza, I hadn't realized how much your core engages when you just put a seatbelt on! But it was a monumental step to have the energy to go out and drive myself. I did okay and realized that while I was doing great at home recuperating, I was not quite ready for a back-to-normal routine. I had a big luncheon for my tennis team, and I was determined to go. I had to drive, talk, and do a bunch of standing and walking around. It was exhausting, but it was progress. From there I went to the surgeon's office for a two-week checkup and he was amazed at how good I looked, how my scars were healing, and all I was able to do.

There are so many more details I could give on this path to my physical recovery. The ups and downs, and the incremental steps back to normal. I was methodical about what I did... from scar-tissue work and scar-reducing moisturizers multiple times a day, to daily abdominal stretching. I brought back my yoga practice piecemeal...small range-of-motion stretching but nothing inverted. I progressed when I was confident I was healed enough. I went back to walking very slowly and incrementally grew in steps and pace, until the routine was back to normal. By the time I got to tennis, six or seven weeks had gone by. John took me out first just to see if I would feel pain when I hit a groundstroke. I was out there with him for an hour and it felt **great**!! Getting to play tennis was the final piece to my physical recovery.

I'm proud of my step-by-step recovery. I am thankful for all the healthy habits I had set up so well beforehand. This is **exactly** how I coach my clients. I encourage them to set the goal and then reverse-engineer it, meaning they work backward and see what they need to do to incrementally reach their goals. Then we figure out the easiest baby steps in that direction. I'll write much more about this later. For now, I'll say that it simply showed me that I had my routines in place. Now, I was building them up slowly to include "all the things" once again post-op. The routine I had developed over the years gave me the steps to know what I needed to get back to: walking, yoga, cardio, and tennis. This will be the focus of this second part of the book. There will be many areas of health and incremental steps for you to take for success in lots of different areas. To put a bow on the topic of my physical healing for now, I'd say I prepared my body and mind to be in the best place possible to receive healing from this surgery. Now, let's get the same for you on your journey of figuring out how to be in your best physical body.

It's just not quite the way it was in our younger days, right? Back when we were young—even when we abused our bodies with what we ate, what we drank, or what we did, we knew that we would recover quickly. Do you remember the times when it wasn't rough on the body back in the day? It's like moving into a new house and you made the move with friends helping and no moving company. It's the same notion as a softball game with friends at the company picnic when you played all out and came home totally sore for the rest of the weekend. This is the weekend-warrior-syndrome, where you think you can do anything, but it's too much because you're sedentary all week. Ah, but as we age, it is a bit different, right? Let's change that shall we? I will offer lots of suggestions for you in Part 3 of this book where I will addresss how to promote habits for well-being. That might be all you need. If you need more, seek an accountability partner. Perhaps hire a health coach. Or find a community with similar goals as yours. There is no need to transform on your own. It can be challenging enough to do without having to rely solely on your willpower. I strongly suggest seeking help in the process.

Chapter 11
Transformational Healing

As I was writing the section above on physical healing, I realized I had been through this very challenging physical and emotional time. Happily, it felt like all my healthcare practices had prepared me to make the most of this situation. I hope it will also guide and serve others to live their best lives, joyfully, even while going through tough, challenging times. And I hope that you will one day be able to see the silver lining in the physically challenging experiences you've been having. While your symptoms and diagnoses may be different from mine, I know that there are life lessons to be gained from all the challenges. I am going to share what I learned. And who knows? Maybe my emotional lessons will speak to you as well.

The first thing I did was to create a space for healing. I cleared my schedule to solely focus on recovery. Interestingly, I became very reflective with all the downtime I had. A lot was brought to my attention from the energy clearing I had six months before when I met with the healer. This cleared the way for me to gain tremendous insight into thoughts and fears that were subconsciously holding me back. I also took a coaching course after my surgery to hone my professional skills. This course turned out to be an enormous unraveling of how and why I show up the way I do. I began to explore my fears. Instead of running away from my fears, I got curious about them. I observed them. I felt them. And most importantly, I embraced them. I found that when I moved toward them and got to the other side, it was less scary. Uncomfortable yes, but I was learning to embrace the discomfort. Don't get me wrong, I certainly prefer to be comfortable, no doubt about that. But I understand that the discomfort is there to teach me something. Breakthrough learning is on the other side of fear. It works to weaken fear. I still feel fearful at times, but I act anyway. What I've noticed lately is that I am acting faster. Calling people out, saying no, letting someone know when I am mad or hurt sooner rather than later. These are situations I was used to sweeping under the rug to avoid conflict or confrontation. This was changing now because my authenticity had become undeniable.

One area of awareness that became blatant was with my relationships. I was immensely grateful for all the love I had in my life—for example, my husband taking amazing care of me, and my friends and family checking in on me daily to let me know they were thinking of me and wishing me well. If you've never recovered from an illness, you may not think about reaching out to people who are healing. Maybe you want them to have space. Maybe you think it is not such a big deal. But surgery **is** a big deal and it is very personal. It's like training for a marathon. Mentally and physically there is a road to travel. You have to prepare and incrementally work to get past milestones in your training. There are milestones in physical healing, too. All triumphs. All important. Having loved ones care enough to witness it with me was heartwarming. They

saw me. They knew it was monumental and because of that, they checked in with me. I viewed each text, phone call, or visit as a testament to their love and care for me. I am beyond blessed and spoiled by my deep friendships and my loving family. Contrastingly, it became quite obvious when someone didn't match up at that level. After the pandemic, and having my two best friends pass away the following year, it became quite clear that each moment is precious. Because of that, I consciously decided to spend time with people who I could have a reciprocal relationship with. I realized that mutually caring relationships are the only types of relationships I want to have.

On a business note, pre-pandemic, I could spend my whole day networking. I could go to a meeting in the morning, meet someone for coffee, and then another person for lunch. It was crazy. Sometimes I would be out of the house all day to meet people who mostly just wanted to sell me their product or service.

I realize now that not every opportunity to network is one I need to take. Same with relationships. Because someone likes me or wants to spend time with me, that doesn't mean I need to say "yes" to giving them my time. Suddenly, in all areas of my life, I became intolerant of being there for other people who were not reciprocating my interest.

In healing, I truly found freedom. My eyes finally opened to who the givers are and who the takers are. I realize that I have no obligation to be "nice" and give my time to people who don't give me value, interest, or care in return.

Do you remember the show *Seinfeld*? There was an episode when the birth control that Elaine used was going out of business. She bought cartons of this contraceptive sponge. With every date she went on, she had to decide if the man was "spongeworthy" or not because there was only a limited supply of the sponges. This is what happens to me now. When deciding if I will give people my time, I now ask myself if they are "spongeworthy enough" to take hours of my time. The greatest reward this awareness has given me is with regard to time. I now know that I can proactively plan my time instead of just reacting to others' requests for my time. It's given me the availability to pursue personal goals and alter business goals to meet my own needs rather than goals suggested by my profession, other people, or society. I also have learned to put myself first. I don't say "yes" to being with people just because they asked. Maybe you already have these great personal boundaries and say "no" to people. But I was raised to be a people pleaser and put others' feelings ahead of my own. So this epiphany was huge for me. In retrospect, it seems so obvious. Spend time with people who show that they value you, and make your goals authentic to the life you want to lead. Doesn't this make sense? Sure. But it wasn't the norm for me. This time for healing from surgery grew into me taking back my life.

Now my days are spent doing 100% of what I want to do. I tend to not have more than a couple of business appointments in a day. I create habits for a healthy, loving lifestyle, which includes a lot of the things I will mention in the next chapter.

I embraced myself and allowed myself space to feel and heal. There is something about being so physically vulnerable that simply opened me up emotionally. I just didn't know I was going to be healing from a lifetime of avoiding uncomfortable emotions. Like everyone else, I had my fair share of hurt and pain. I've spent most of my life looking on the bright side and not dwelling in the past. What I realized is that my emotional fears were based on imprints I've had from circumstances in my past, so looking at them was very helpful in releasing current fears because they were all made up in my head from stories I had unconsciously been telling myself. Recognizing that everything we think is made up, I thought if I am going to make up stories, I might as well make them to benefit me instead of holding me back. Right?

I have learned to trust my instincts more. I learned this in my physical healing by not rushing and, instead, going at a pace that would serve my recovery. I have learned to trust my instincts emotionally and be true to my most authentic self.

Grieving the loss of Randy and Erica, both friends for about fifty years, rocked me to my core. These two knew me like no others. They loved every morsel of my body, mind, and soul. They always had hours to talk to me about every minute detail of my life. I can't describe in words how thankful I am to have had them in my life. Needless to say, physical healing provided me with the time to feel my sadness, an emotion I was not used to experiencing. Now, interestingly, I embrace sadness because it is an actual comfort to me. It was and continues to be a reconnecting experience. I reconnect to them. Very few people know what I lost. But at some time we all experience loss. As you may already know, most people do not continually check in on you about how your grieving is going. Maybe they think grieving ends. Maybe it's the lack of conversation around death in our culture. I guess it can be considered a morbid topic. To me, it's not morbid, it's a comfort. Being sad brings me closer to them. It reminds me of what I lost. It is a comfort to still be connected to them in some way.

Why do I share about my emotional healing in a book about digestive issues?

I want you to be ready for anything that may come up.

I want you to be open.

Healing a physical wound can simply be the guide to get you to heal from wounds that have been there long before any physical ailment developed. I strongly suggest taking the time to process whatever may come up for you. Allow healing at any level that presents itself to you.

The purpose of the next part of this book is to equip you with foundational habits of health that I cultivated for myself. It is my desire that by employing some or all of these habits, you will feel, heal, and thrive in any situation. Sounds good? Of course it does!

Let's take a look at this next part of the book and get started on how you can be the dominant force in your own life. You can learn how to instill habits that will help you thrive. Imagine that.

Part 3

Habits to Promote Wellbeing

It is our birthright to live a happy, fulfilled life. So many of us are creating lives that do not serve us well. What if we created a path to healing, freedom, and joy? I know it's possible because I'm living that life. I want to share with you what I know. Simple tweaks in your daily routines to establish a foundation of positivity that can lead to great health, a positive mindset, and a zest for living in the moment. Let's start by delving into this idea of habit formation.

Chapter 12
Why Create a Habit

One aspect of my life that got me through the physical and emotional healing were the habits I cultivated over the decades. I want to spend ample time on this part of the book because this is where most people can use guidance. Whether or not you even have digestive issues, these habits will optimize your overall health and therefore be good for your digestion, too. Developing healthy habits will not eliminate all medical conditions—such was the case with me. I had a gallstone almost the same size as my gallbladder. There were not many other options to cure my attacks other than removing the gallbladder. I do feel that I lasted ten years with the gallstone because my healthy habits made my body so healthy that I was able to lessen the amount of pain and the frequency of the attacks because I wasn't feeding it foods that would bring on an attack. Because I was trying to figure things out naturally through internet research, I developed lots of healthy behaviors that made my body a better environment to avoid attacks. Even though I didn't really know what was going on, I made healthy choices based on the suggestions for the symptoms I was experiencing.

There are so many reasons for establishing good habits. Granted, I am focused on digestive issues because that is the topic of this book. You picked up the book to help yourself cope with the years of digestive issues you have been experiencing, right? I am here to say that for **any** goal you have, you will need to build habits to help achieve them. For me, writing this, my very first book, I had to create book-writing behaviors and habits to accomplish my goal of writing it. To be successful in life, you need structure. I tell my clients that structure is their friend. My whole career goal as a health coach is to help people replace behaviors that do not serve them and replace them with behaviors that will help them reach their goals... whatever their goals are. While I predominantly help people lose weight, the habits we build include eating throughout the day, drinking water, and getting sufficient sleep. The list goes on. But we take **one habit** at a time and build each habit up so that it becomes brainless and takes little effort to accomplish. Think back to when you were learning how to brush your teeth. You needed a lot of help with the toothpaste, with how much time to brush, and perhaps other things. At first, probably a parent was helping you and you slowly learned to do more and more of it on your own until you were brushing your teeth on your own. Fast-forward to the current day. You brush your teeth twice a day with no help. The thought of needing help is comical because you mastered it a long time ago. Brushing your teeth is brainless. It is automatic. You could do it with your eyes closed. You do it in the morning and in the evening without much thought. You don't need any reminders. You just get it done automatically.

This is the same with achieving any goal. Weight loss is multifaceted, so I will often ask a client which is the easiest habit of all the parts to create health and lose weight. Then we start there with the easiest piece of the puzzle. Why start with the easiest part? Well, self-esteem and negative self-talk have a lot to do with the answer. As humans, we tend to have our minds programmed negatively. Of the 70,000 thoughts we have in a day, about 80% of them are negative. Oh my goodness, that's not a good thing. This negative self-talk is generally telling ourselves why we can't do things. Imagine our own worst critic allowed in such a sacred place as our minds. Yikes. I suggest that we build a case to prove to our inner critic that it is wrong. There are many ways to combat this negative voice. One way I encourage my clients to do so is to start with a behavior change that is so small that accomplishing it is almost a certainty. They could get it done even as their head was hitting the pillow before bedtime. This allows your brain to say, "Wow, I did what I said I was going to do. Wow. I kept the promise to myself." Then trust begins to form, and maybe for the first time, you believe in yourself. You believe that you can reach the goal you set because it's not even that hard. This will be my focus in the upcoming sections of the book: to help you choose behaviors that you can begin to solidify without much effort. Just like brushing your teeth is a habit to keep your dental health, I will address many types of habits and you can choose which ones will help you move forward for your overall health. It's always best to work with a coach, or at least an accountability partner. We will talk about the value of accountability in Chapter 20. For now, I strongly suggest trying one new habit at a time. I would not suggest trying to implement all of the suggestions at the same time. The upcoming suggestions are meant to create sustainable, lifelong changes. As long as you are incrementally moving forward, that is what is important. This is not a boot camp mentality where you go all out for thirty days and then go back to your old, bad habits. While there's a time and place for boot camps, I believe in giving ourselves grace at every opportunity. This is our life. I do not see the benefit of beating ourselves up in an attempt to move closer to our goals. I believe in living a joyful life whereby improvement, and working towards goals are woven into daily life. The **process** is what needs to be celebrated rather than simply celebrating results. Sure, we are all working towards results and that is noble. However, it is ok to get where we want to go and be kind to ourselves along the way. That is the premise of the book. We are works in progress. As a work in progress, we don't ever "arrive." It's silly then, to live a whole life being mad at ourselves for not being "there" yet. Right?

So let's read on. Decide what feels best to pursue and try that first. This book is designed for you to pick up anytime you need momentum or guidance in establishing and maintaining a new habit. Let's see what options are laid out for you.

Chapter 13
Morning Routine

Most people start their day by rolling over groggily in bed and reaching for their phone before they even go to the bathroom. Are you one of them? What do you look at first? Email? Texts? Stocks? Social media? Sports results? I try not to do this. It's a challenge for me, especially if I need my phone for my alarm. I turn off the alarm and then inevitably something catches my eye, like a text or something, and bam! I'm on my phone before I start my optimal morning routine. Has this happened to you as well? You wake up from a peaceful sleep and all of a sudden, your emotions can be hijacked by a text asking you to do something immediately, or a social media post that intrigues you.

After this foray into the wide world of navigating all that your phone has to offer, you realize it's getting late. Sound familiar? So you rush around trying to get dressed and grab a cup of coffee, a donut if you're lucky. Then run out the door, hoping to get to work on time. In a half-assed frenzy, you start to stress because your boss already complained about the number of times you've walked in late... and so your days begin. Would you agree that this is not an ideal way to start the day? Rushed, stressed, and off to a bad start is the opposite of how you want to start a day if you're looking to be your optimal self.

The way you start your morning sets the tone for how your whole day will go. Getting into habits that can boost your mood can help improve the productivity and the pleasantness of each and every day. Imagine being able to actually plan to have a good day. It is possible. Let's take a closer look at some behavior options we all have available to us to create fabulous days for ourselves.

A morning routine that serves your best self is what I suggest. May McCarthy, in her book, *The Path To Wealth*, writes about meeting with your chief spiritual officer, your CSO, each morning. She explains that many executives have a morning meeting with their whole C-suite to get direction and guidance to make the day stay on track, maximize time, and opportunity. This author suggests having this type of meeting with yourself each morning. Get in touch with your highest self. How do you want to feel? What is the most important thing to accomplish today? Is it in a relationship? Business? Self-care practices? All of the above? It's a check-in. Before all the craziness of the day begins, it's a centering process to keep you focused throughout the day on what's most important to you. Even if you get off track, you have your morning meeting to reflect on and get you back to what is meaningful to you, to your authentic self... not just busy stuff and putting out fires.

The morning "meeting" can take many shapes and forms. It's almost like an empowerment routine. You can exercise, journal, meditate, shower, pray, plan, hydrate, and do anything else that lifts the individual emotionally, spiritually, educationally, or physically.

Personally, my morning routine includes three things: meditation, journaling, and reading. If all goes well, that lasts about an hour and I am ready to start my day. I feel centered, grounded, and spiritual after meditating. Meditation gives me a peaceful start to my day. Journaling helps me to express my challenges and triumphs. It is like having a therapy session with my highest self. And reading awakens me to other ideas, other lives, and other places.

All three parts of my morning routine are based on lots of research and studies on what successful people do to start their days. You can, of course, choose which elements you'd like to include for yourself based on what would serve you best to create the most intentional and purposeful start to your day. Let's delve into one of my favorite parts of my morning routine first: meditation.

Chapter 14
Meditation

Why Is Meditation Important?

No longer is meditation viewed as something that only spiritual healers and hippies do. Meditation improves both physical and mental well-being. Meditation can lower blood pressure, boost your immune system, reduce stress and anxiety, and improve sleep, just to name a few. Isn't that amazing? I wish people would take to meditating instead of having a glass of wine to relax.

I know some people who say that they "can't" meditate; they say they don't know how to still their minds or keep it quiet. To which I usually reply, "that it is because you are human." Our minds tend to keep going. It's not necessary to still the mind completely to get all the benefits from the practice of meditating. I liken the misconception about what meditation is to the word or concept of God. I used to be uncomfortable with using the word *God*, because I wasn't sure if what I meant by *God* was the same meaning held by the other person in my conversation. Most of my life I just avoided the word, or I got used to using words and terms like *the Universe*, *Mother Nature*, or *a higher power*. Now, I'm clear on what I mean by it, and I am not so concerned anymore on whether someone understands my concept of God or not.

Meditation carries the same misconceptions. Some people think it is one thing, and others think differently. I want to dispel the beliefs about what meditation is. There are as many definitions as there are practices. Meaning that everyone can meditate in very different ways. You can do what feels best to you. Simple deep breathing is a form of meditation. Listening to a guided meditation on YouTube would suffice. You can take workshops and classes to learn from other experts in the various genres of meditation. Here is a link to a free meditation that I offer on my website: (www.MyCoachSue.com/meditation). You can start there. I would be honored to start your meditation journey with you.

What Habits to Start With

Knowing the massive benefits that come to our bodies and minds when we meditate, I bet you are eager to try it yourself.

Let's talk about you specifically. Where are you? Are you one of the people who think that you could never meditate? Do you already incorporate deep breathing in your day? Do you meditate sometimes? Or do you want to add time or depth to a practice you have already established? Your answers to these questions will determine where you need to start. My expertise is starting with the novice, so that is where I will begin here.

How to Form the Habits

What I always suggest, and you'll see it as a common theme as we go through all the healthy habits, is to start with a micro-goal, or a tiny habit. Your big goal may be to meditate for twenty minutes each day. I suggest to my clients something more in the neighborhood of one minute. Yes, that's right, one minute. Maybe it would be sitting with your eyes closed for one minute, or just taking ten deep breaths each day. You may say, "Yes, but Coach Sue, that is nowhere near my goal," to which I would reply "that's ok." The goal when beginning a new habit is to make it as easy as possible to create the space for the larger habit down the road. Once the easy habit is implemented, clients then feel proud and confident that they did what they said they would do. They build trust with themselves that they did what they said they would do, after years, perhaps, of letting themselves down when they have tried so many times before to improve their health to no avail. This is why working with a coach can be so beneficial. They can help you plan the smallest, easiest steps to take to help you build up to your macro, or bigger goal. In time, this helps to create sustainability and a stable platform from which you can continually add more micro, or tiny habits to reach your ultimate and ever growing goals. If you feel like the habit is ridiculously small and easy, you're on the right track.

I will share an example of implementing a meditation habit with one of my clients. I'll call her Sharon. Sharon is the CEO of a big company. She is a great time manager, juggling motherhood, corporate responsibilities, running a household, and working to improve her health and reduce stress. She has many things to do in a day and she didn't feel that she could squeeze in one more task into her highly structured day. However, she really wanted to reduce the amount of stress her body was absorbing from her endlessly busy days. Sharon was willing to start with a one-minute micro habit. First, we established a chair in her bedroom that we designated as her meditation chair. Her first goal was to simply sit in it for one minute each day. That's it. Sit still. Eyes closed. No agenda. That's it. She set an alarm for one minute. She could spend more time in the meditation chair if she wanted to, but the goal was one minute. This was a habit that even if she had the busiest day on the planet (which most days were for her), she could do this right before bed. Needless to say Sharon was a champ at sitting in her chair and keeping her eyes closed for one minute. When we had a coaching call after one week, she said that she was starting to look forward to this time and was even extending it to a few minutes because it was so relaxing. She realized it was the only time she stopped all day long. It was a rest. She told me how she noticed her mind whirling when she sat down and thoughts from throughout the day were bubbling up. This was a keen observation. So we decided to play around with that. I gave her an optional activity. It was to watch those thoughts. See them as objects. Even imagine them like clouds and watch the thoughts float by. The conversations she had in the conference room that day... acknowledge them, then watch them float by. And do that with each following thought. This was proving to be more of a challenge for her. I reminded her that it's ok to get stuck on a thought. After all, we are human and thinking is what makes us human. Nonetheless, she was getting frustrated that she could only see the thoughts float by sometimes. So we tried another meditative experience. While she was in the meditation chair, she would focus on her breathing. She practiced meditation in her coaching session while we were together. I told her to close her eyes and notice her breath. To pay attention to her breath in and her breath out. Then I asked her a few questions: How does it feel? Does your belly fill up with air as you breathe in? Is air coming out of your mouth or your nose as you exhale? I asked Sharon to open her eyes and tell me what she noticed. She told me:

> "I was very focused on my breathing."
> "My belly was going in and out more deliberately than ever before."
> "Taking deep breaths felt very intentional."
> "I only thought about your voice and breathing."
> "It was like watching my body breathe."
> "I was in control of my breathing while I was observing it."
> To which I replied, "That is meditation!"

What hit home for Sharon, and I hope for you as well, is that meditation is not necessarily the absence of thought, but rather the redirection of thought. It is being the observer of thought and of oneself. Meditation is a personal journey and everyone's experience is different. If this type of practice is important for you to incorporate into your daily life, take a gentle approach. Start with a tiny micro-habit and observe the benefits. Once you experience enhanced well-being, you will be a fan and you'll do what it takes to incorporate this new habit into your daily life...even if it winds up only being for a minute! Remember that consistency is key. Over time you may gradually increase the duration, and explore different techniques or types of meditations that resonate with you.

Chapter 15
Movement

Why Movement is Important

Movement has important benefits for both the body and the mind. Here are some of the main benefits:

1. Movement helps strengthen the heart, allowing it to pump blood more efficiently, thus lowering the risk of heart disease.
2. Movement can help burn calories and maintain a healthy weight, reducing the risk of obesity and other digestive issues.
3. Weight-bearing exercises can actually help build and maintain bone density, reducing the risk of osteoporosis.
4. Regular movement can lower the risk of chronic diseases such as diabetes, hypertension, and certain types of cancer!!

5. Movement has been shown to reduce symptoms of depression and anxiety and improve overall mood and mental wellbeing.
6. Regular movement can improve physical endurance and energy levels, making it easier to perform daily activities and reduce fatigue.
7. Movement can help improve the quality and duration of sleep.
8. Movement has been shown to improve memory, focus, and attention.
9. Increased lifespan!!

Whoa. Those are amazing benefits. Sign me up to move more. Don't you want to get up and move right now?

What Habits to Start With

Oh my goodness, there are so many places you can start. The starting point depends on what your current activity level is and what your goals are. I have my clients track their activity to assess where they are. Many clients will say they never exercise and it is overwhelming to think of a routine that doesn't sound daunting to them. Oftentimes the easiest thing for them to start tracking is steps. Most people already have devices, watches, or apps that track their steps. This gives insight into where to start goal setting. If a client has a small number of steps each day, an attainable micro-habit could be to increase the steps by just 500-1000 over their average baseline. Clients are often shocked at how many steps they take in a day. They think they are inactive because they don't have an exercise routine, when in fact they have lots of movement each day; they just never categorized it as exercise.

Let me pause here to make an important distinction between movement and exercise for the express purpose of improving your health. Exercise is considered the "E word" with most of my clients. They dread it. Movement, however, can be anything you do using your body. If we want sustainable change in the area of exercise, it's important to create a lifestyle that is not sedentary. The body is meant to move and to do hard things. But life nowadays is pretty easy on the body, with drive-thrus, remote controls, and Amazon delivering a lot of our packages. We used to get movement in by just going to the store. Daily movement is mostly gone. Between work and a life of many conveniences, we are not moving much on a normal day. What's great about starting with something as simple as steps is that it is great data. When you see how many steps you are currently taking, then you can make a small goal to improve. When you just start moving, you'll amazingly want to do more. I have one client so motivated to move that even though her microhabit was to just add five minutes of movement in her routine in a day, she found herself dancing every morning, walking the dog daily, making a step goal of 10,000 steps, and adding twenty minutes on her exercise bike. One good energetic move in a day leads to another. I do suggest growing your routine incrementally so you create a sustainable habit that will become the foundation for the next one. In the case of the client I just mentioned, although she increased her activity quickly, she found joy in all she did. That's the point. If you are not finding joy, rather you are feeling like the movement is arduous or boring, I suggest starting somewhere else. Habit implementation is not about gritting your teeth and bearing it.

It is about creating a joyful space whereby more arduous tasks are welcome down the road.

After I healed enough from my gall-bladder-removal surgery, I did not immediately get back to my fast-paced, three-to-four-mile walks. I had to start all over. I started with one slow walk around a half-mile loop and that was almost too much for me. I waited another week, and then I was able to walk slowly around the half-mile loop twice. I gradually got back to my regular walking routine. I was thankful I had established this routine because it gave me guideposts in my healing. I had a routine I was incrementally working to get back to. For those of you just starting with a movement/exercise routine, let's delve into how to establish these habits in the next section.

How to Form the Habits

Have you heard of the term *reverse engineering*? Simply put, reverse engineering is envisioning the end goal and figuring out what is required of you to get there. If you want to run a marathon but have never run a mile, running a mile may be a starting point. With this goal in particular, there are many apps, personal trainers, and gyms that will help you build routines to give you the workouts and training schedule to get you there within a desired time range. Perhaps your macro-goal is to workout five days a week and you are not exercising at all. You may start with one day a week. You may say, "Sue, one day a week is a lame goal; I can do more than that." To which I would say, "Great. Do more. But know that you are a success if you meet your first micro-goal." In other words, you are a winner if you only exercise once a week because that is the micro-habit. If you want to do more, do more. I want your initial goal to be so easy that you can 100% get it done. Once you have established that, create another goal. Perhaps two days a week, and so on until you achieve your macro-goal of exercising five days a week.

When I was building the habit of stretching into my routine, I knew my ultimate goal was to stretch twenty minutes every day. My micro-habit was to stretch for **one minute**! Yep, that's all. I set up a routine of going to our upstairs family room, getting my mat out, and putting music on. Generally, I stretched for five minutes, but if I felt rushed, or not in the mood to stretch, I recorded stretching for even one minute as a win.

Why such tiny habits? It breeds confidence and trust that you are doing what you said you would do. This confidence and trust are huge. In my line of work, clients are wanting to lose weight. By the time they get to me, they have tried so many diets and have failed to lose it all or keep it off. I see that they have lost the trust in themselves to accomplish their goals. This mindset is what thwarts the desire to try to implement healthy routines because they expect to fail. Breaking down a giant goal into small baby steps is a way to build self-esteem and confidence while reaching new goals.

Tammy, one of my weight-loss clients, had kept the weight off for a couple of years. Making healthy food choices had become the norm for her. She was now ready to dive into the exercise piece of her healthy routine. She had pretty much stopped exercising in a gym since the pandemic. She was walking and doing some exercise videos, but she was ready to get more serious about a structured exercise plan that included strength training. Tammy joined a local gym. Her goal was to lift weights two days a week. She already included cardio in her weekly routine and was looking to strengthen and grow muscle mass. She hired a personal trainer once a month for general instruction and accountability. Going to the gym was not part of her normal activity, so at first the goal was to go to the gym one day a week. Tammy started with a yoga class, an aqua class, belly dancing, and the sauna—in no particular order. All valuable activities for varying reasons, but not quite specific to her goal. The reason we made her first micro-habit simply going to the gym was to get gym time in her schedule and have her feel good about it. It was fun for her to do all those things. After a few weeks, she had her first session with her trainer where she learned how to use the equipment. She then began to incorporate weight training once a week. Tammy added the second day at the gym once weightlifting was affixed to her weekly schedule. Occasionally she would throw in the second day of weight training. Now several months down the road, Tammy is going to the gym twice a week and weightlifting both times. She sees her trainer monthly to get suggestions on what muscle group to incorporate and gets help on developing routines that will gradually get her the percentage of muscle mass she is looking to develop. It may have taken Tammy more months than most people want to wait, but she has a routine that she built gradually and can maintain. That's the key element here: sustainability.

Many of us have seen what happens when a new membership is bought at a gym. The gym is usually packed with New Year's resolutioners in January—and only in January —then it goes back to just the long-time members. Why is this so often the case? Well, this is a multi-faceted answer, which could vary for every person, but basically it goes to motivation. Many people lose motivation quickly without accountability. Sometimes new gym members expect to see results immediately, and that is not usually the case. People go in with gung-ho ambition, exercising to extremes, then feeling sore and in pain. This type of rigor is not sustainable in a long-term manner. If you feel lots of pain after each exercise session to the point of not being able to walk, would you be motivated to go back again for another workout?

In closing this section on how to create a movement or exercise goal, the secret is to start with the end in mind. Break it down to the smallest first step you can think of and start there. Do that consistently and then add another baby step until you've reached your ultimate exercise goal. You'll be amazed at how sustainable these routines will become. Surprisingly, a nice side effect will be the continual planning of what your next goal will be. You will continually look to become a better version of yourself. This is another reason why you want to enjoy the journey. The destination never arrives. It is always a journey. Let's enjoy the trip. Baby steps allow us to celebrate more often. Feeling good, accomplishing goals, and improving your health all at the same time is amazing. It's a win/win/win for you.

Chapter 16

Hydration

Why Hydration is Important

The benefits to keeping hydrated are innumerable. Before I give you a partial list of them, let me tell you a little story that will spotlight one of the reasons why hydration is so important. I often give a free consultation to potential clients to see if we are a fit for each other. I had one of these calls with a woman I know from a locally based social media group. After asking her a few questions, it was evident that she did not drink any water. She drank fruit juice and sweet tea all day. She was not ready to hire me but I asked if it was okay to give her a tip to help her get closer to her goal of losing forty pounds. So I suggested the tiniest of improvements, which was to replace just one of her sweet beverages each day with an eight-ounce glass of water. I said to her that if she wanted a bigger challenge, a goal of drinking a minimum of sixty-four ounces of water is a great target to aim for, but beginning with one glass of water per day is a good place to start. And she was on her way. About a month and a half later, I saw a social media post she made. She was celebrating losing fifteen pounds. She gave me a shout out. She wrote that she replaced all her sweet drinks with water. She took my advice—she took the bigger challenge, and implemented a foundational habit that will assist in reaching her goals. While drinking plenty of water is great for weight loss, you're not going to believe how medicinal it is. Here is a long, and non-exhaustive list.

1. It prevents dehydration.
2. It flushes out toxins.
3. It clears the complexion.
4. It heals dull skin.
5. It prevents chapped lips.
6. It aids in weight loss. It's zero calories.
7. It increases metabolism.
8. It aids digestion.
9. It relieves headaches.
10. It regulates body temperature.
11. It boosts the immune system.
12. It increases energy.
13. It maximizes workouts.
14. It regulates kidney function.
15. It prevents kidney stones.
16. It reduces hangover symptoms.
17. It increases brain function.
18. It improves mood.
19. It elevates alertness.
20. It fights high blood pressure.
21. It protects joints.
22. It relieves congestion.
23. It decreases the risk of heartburn.
24. It improves heart health.

25. It maintains pH balance.
26. It prevents osteoporosis.
27. It aids breathing. (Your body naturally loses water when you breathe.)
28. It improves body functions, including digestion!
29. It treats backaches. Water helps cushion your joints!
30. It fights bladder infections.
31. It improves the ability to think.
32. It relieves fatigue.
33. It transports nutrients throughout your body.
34. It serves as an appetite suppressant.
35. It reduces the symptoms of asthma.
36. It prevents premature wrinkles.
37. It fights tooth decay.
38. It beats bad breath.

Need I say anything else about why drinking water is so important? Every organ and system in your body operates better by being hydrated. Let's figure out if you are getting enough water in your day, and what habits you can implement to be sure your hydration needs are being met. This is what the next section is aimed at helping you with.

What Habits to Start With

Before you know where to start, you need to know where you are. So my first question to you is, how many ounces of water do you drink now? If you do not know how much you drink daily, your first task is to track your water intake for a week. There are so many apps you can use to track water. Or, of course, old-fashioned paper and pen would work well, too!

After tracking the number of ounces you drink on an average day, we'll see a baseline, or an average daily consumption amount. When you know how much you drink, you may find that your hydration is perfect. Some people aim for sixty-four ounces a day, some aim for half their body weight in ounces. For example, I weigh 160 pounds. My goal is to drink eighty ounces of water each day, which is half my body weight in ounces. You can consult with your health professional if you would like some guidance in making a decision about how many ounces of water is in your best interest to drink.

How to Form the Habits

If we want to make this hydration habit a brainless habit, then we need to be strategic in setting it up. This is a great time to introduce to you the strategy of habit stacking. Habit stacking is where you attach a new habit to a habit that is rock solid. Think about several habits that happen every day, at least 99% of the time. For you, that may mean making coffee in the morning, brushing your teeth, arriving at work, watching TV, or making the bed. Take a moment to think about, and write down a list of habits that are strongholds in your daily life. Go ahead and make that list right now, at least mentally.

Let's say you make coffee for yourself each morning. You could put a bottle of water by the coffee maker at night, so that in the morning, when your coffee is brewing, you can drink a bottle of water. You set up the cue, or reminder by placing the bottle of water by the coffee machine before the morning comes. This reminds you of your goal to drink more and gives you time to drink it while the coffee is brewing. Coffee in the morning is rock solid. That's why pairing it, or stacking another habit with it is a good idea.

Another common habit-stacking time is before or after brushing your teeth. Most people brush their teeth at least twice a day, giving plenty of opportunities to pair that habit with water drinking. You just have to set up the environment for success. In this case, that means getting water bottles to the bathroom where you brush your teeth and have it placed near the toothbrush to act as a cue or reminder to drink either before or after your brush. Soon the habit of drinking a bottle of water will be paired with teeth-brushing time.

One more example would be TV watching. I assume many of you are streaming some show each night or watching cable TV. If this is one of your daily habits, perhaps you can put a bottle of water by the remote, or simply put a sticky note by the place you watch TV. Perhaps your goal is to drink after each show eventually. At the beginning it is about making space for drinking water when you are on the couch. Once you get that behavior paired with TV watching, you can progress to more quantity and frequency. It may seem like you are only taking baby steps and it can feel insignificant. Let me tell you, baby steps are hugely significant. You progress at a pace that feels effortless, yet you are moving incrementally toward your goals. It's as if you only have one task to do all day, you know you can get it done.

Aside from habit stacking, two fun ways to install hydration habits are to buy a fun water bottle so you get some pleasure from using it and choose hydrating drinks such as herbal tea, sparkling water, mineral water, or coconut water. Caffeinated drinks and sugary drinks are not hydrating, so they don't count. Having a variety of beverage choices can be motivating. I usually have alkaline water, lemon water, coconut water, vitamin water, and herbal tea each day to keep me from just drinking plain water all day. Will you mix up different types of water? Or are you good with plain water throughout the day?

Whichever game plan you choose, start right now to give your body the water it needs to work best. Bottoms up, everyone!!

Chapter 17
Sleep

Millions of Americans are sleep-deprived. Are you one of them? Have you ever not gotten all the sleep you needed? Were you tired? Cranky? Irritable? Hungry? Ineffective? Those are just some of the side effects of lack of sleep. If you are not getting all the sleep you need on a regular basis, the body and the mind cannot function optimally. I'll share a couple of examples of clients I have worked with to illustrate some of the setbacks that can occur.

One of my clients, Joann, was doing everything right in her weight-loss journey but was getting little return on her good choices. She was eating well, hydrating, and exercising. When I questioned her about her sleep she said it was horrible. She rarely slept through the night. I figured this was most likely her stumbling block. Our bodies are so amazing. Get this: if you don't have enough sleep, your body produces more of the hormone called ghrelin, which increases appetite. Simultaneously, it produces less of the hormone leptin, which normally gives a feeling of satiation. Basically, without enough sleep we are hungrier. And it's not our fault. It's just how the body works. If we get enough sleep, those hormones turn around and naturally produce more leptin and less ghrelin. Amazing, right?

After Joann learned about this reversal of hormones, she immediately saw the benefit in prioritizing her sleep and she went right to work setting up new behaviors to encourage a better quality of sleep.

Every part of your body needs rest, even your bowels. If your bowels have insufficient rest and muscle fatigue, they will have difficulty pushing out the waste they are meant to naturally rid you of. I was working with another client, Laurie, on solidifying her habits to improve her overall health. We started with good food choices. She was eating fruits and vegetables, legumes, and whole grains. One would think she would have regular bowel movements, but she didn't. When she told me that she was getting only a few hours of sleep because her shift at work changed, it all made sense. Cortisol and melatonin are hormones that get released based on what time of day it is. More cortisol during the day keeps us awake and alert. Melatonin, which makes us sleepy, is released at night. There's not much you can do to change your schedule if your job has you working swing or graveyard shifts, which is very common here in Las Vegas. These shifts are popular among casino workers and nurses. Laurie is a nurse. There isn't anything she could do about her work schedule. We looked at what she did have control over. Her hours were from 4:00 p.m. to midnight. When she got home from work she would get some chores done and then relax. Her goal was to create a ritual, or schedule, that would promote quality sleep. She wanted to be in bed by 3:00 a.m. She slept until 11:00 a.m. This wake-up time gave her the sleep she needed and plenty of time to do errands, exercise and all the other things one has to do in life...even meeting friends for lunch in the middle of the week. Did it solve her constipation issues? It certainly did. In a short time after installing a new sleep ritual, Laurie was getting solid, restorative sleep and her days of constipation were behind her. I remind my clients, as I will tell you now, that I am not a medical professional and if they have **any** condition, even constipation that is persistent, they need to see their physician. Improving sleep habits is an excellent way to be proactive in your health journey, but it is not a replacement for medical attention. Remember that. Moving on, there are so many medicinal benefits to a good night's sleep. Let's take a look at some more reasons why sleep is so valuable.

Why Sleep is Important

Getting enough sleep can help you:

- Get sick less often
- Stay at a healthy weight
- Lower your risk for serious health problems, like diabetes and heart disease
- Reduce stress and improve your mood
- Think more clearly and do better in school and at work
- Get along better with people
- Make good decisions and avoid injuries—for example, drowsy drivers cause thousands of car accidents every year

The list goes on. Sleep is nature's nurse in so many ways. There is an endless list of how sleep benefits the body and the mind. Above are some of these highlights. There is a range of what's considered a healthy amount of sleep depending on your age. Most research points to seven hours or more as a sufficient amount for adults. There are so many variables involved such as sleep disorders, work schedules, and whether you feel well-rested when you wake up. I would suggest seeing your physician if you do not sleep well—not necessarily for medication, but to get a diagnosis, if there is one to make. For example, I understand that if insomnia is an issue, medication may provide sleep, thus allowing the body and brain to get some temporary rest. Sleep medication does not provide a deep, restful sleep, however, and alternative behaviors will need to come into play. Perhaps the self-care section coming up could offer some suggestions to help with better sleep, too. Not all sleep issues are related to stress levels, but if they are, the self-care section may be of help. Suffice it to say, sleep is an important habit to cultivate. I'll share some habits for you to choose from so that you can institute the ones that make sense for you. Experiment with them to see which help you to get the quality sleep that you need.

What Habits to Start With

It's tough for me to tell you which habit to start with because the answer will be different for every person depending on what their sleep goal is and also what their current habits are. What I do know is that the good ole reverse-engineering model is the place to look and then decide what is ideal for you. Reverse-engineering, again, means to start with the end in mind, then backtrack to find steps to help you achieve the goal. Do you need to get more hours of sleep? Do you need to get a better quality of sleep? Do you have trouble falling asleep, or staying asleep? Your situation makes all the difference in where you begin. Take a minute right now to decide what your sleep challenge is. Although, I am guessing you are well aware.

When I take on new clients who want to lose weight, or have any other health concerns, I ask about their sleep patterns and evening time routines. After discussing their sleep habits, the most common obstacles with sleep are staying up too late or not being able to fall asleep. Let's take a look at those situations with a health-coaching eye.

Staying Up Late

The simple answer is go to bed earlier, right? It's just not that easy for those who have a lot to do before bedtime to make their careers or households thrive. So we start with a micro-habit. Can you come up with some ideas for a micro-habit? Remember it has to be tiny, and doable.

Here's one suggestion; go to bed ONE minute earlier!

For me, I know that if I go to bed at 11:30 or later, I will be tired the next day. The ideal time for me is 10:00-10:30 p.m. When I am following my healthy habits (which is definitely not every single day), I make sure to finish up what I'm doing by 10:00 p.m. Then I head upstairs, which signals my mind to get into bedtime ritual mode. I won't go through all the little things I do before bed, but suffice it to say, I have a routine. This routine now tells my brain and my body that bedtime is nearing. It is no different from when we train infants to sleep at night. They are not born with a circadian rhythm. We train babies to sleep by creating a bedtime ritual. Maybe the indoor house lights are dimmed. Then there is an evening bath, an evening feeding, a bedtime story, and laying down in the crib. The parent is setting up the environment for the baby to learn what to do in that crib. There is a winding-down process—a process I notice many adults are not that great at implementing. Many stay up late doing things, whether it is watching TV, folding laundry, writing a book, or a myriad of other reasons. If we can create a micro-habit of just one minute earlier, we are creating new brain space for the habit that can eventually grow larger once we get it started! Your brain will amaze you. It will look for ways to end your evening earlier! I will give you some suggestions in the next section, though.

Not being able to fall asleep

Some people cannot fall asleep due to body aches and pains. Some people have an active mind, and for this reason it is a challenge to fall asleep. Let's take a look at the busy mind. How do we slow it down enough to fall asleep in a timely manner? Let's take a look at Cheryl, one of my clients who had this exact issue. She is a CEO of a large company, and a mom of three school-age kids. She has to make the most of every moment so that she can function at work at an executive level. She also wants to make family life a priority, which means spending time with the kids in the evening on most nights. She has a cooperative husband who shares cooking, shopping, and laundry but still has those tasks on her mind as she shares in the home responsibilities. They have help from a cleaning service, and they order groceries online and either pick them up or get them delivered. Cheryl is task-centered and gets all the things done or delegates them. In any case, she runs a well-oiled machine. The issue is she has no down time in a day. She is constantly making decisions in the moment and has no time to slow it down. When bedtime arrives, she lays awake processing all that has happened in the day and thinks of what needs to be done the next day.

This is another example of where we can apply a reverse-engineering process. I asked Cheryl how she could "mind dump" during the day without taking too much time from her day. The answer we came up with was journaling. We started her with a journal at work. In the journal she put wins for the day, challenges during the day, items she would come back the next day to immediately work on first thing in the morning, and then her top three most important things to get done after that. She had this list to look at as soon as she got to the office, which was also a time saver. This was working wonders and she was falling asleep much faster. Later on she added a journal for home and personal life, which followed the same format: wins for the day, challenges, and what three things would be her top priority for her own self care and her family time each evening. The journaling acts as a release, a reflection, and an honest look at the day. When she would reflect and celebrate her wins at work and at home, it helped her to realize how much she accomplished each and every day. Whereas before the journal, it was endless worrying about if she did enough, which sadly tends to translate to feeling like you are not enough. With the journaling process, not only did she celebrate her wins, but she also navigated challenges and had them figured out enough to keep them off of her mind when at home. In essence, she was more satisfied and therefore more relaxed with increased self-esteem. What amazing results for implementing one tiny journaling habit. Of course, there are many alternative behaviors you can come up with to help get your mind rested enough for sleep. You can probably guess, given my discussion of meditation earlier in the book, that I love that as a solution for sleep challenges, too. Here I wanted to give you Cheryl's solution because it can have a big impact with just a small investment. Basically you get a restful mind by getting it all out on paper. I suggested to Cheryl that she go out and buy a fun pen and a pretty journal so it helped her to look forward to doing the journal entries. It totally worked for her and she now has her own school-aged children journaling their wins and challenges for the day as well. It has become a win for the whole family. In a day and age when mental health awareness is at a peak, it's great to have these self-care practices in place to solidify our own mental health. We all know that it is difficult to have good mental health without good sleep. This practice was a win for Cheryl and her whole family.

How to Form the Habits

Now that we have a specific goal, we can work on cultivating one tiny habit at a time. We want to prompt the goal to happen naturally by setting ourselves up for success. Just like the dedicated parent who creates a sleep routine for the baby, let's get you to parent yourself. If you need more sleep, you have to go to bed earlier. In order to go to bed earlier you have to stop what you are doing earlier, even if it is just one minute. One idea is to set an alarm to give you enough time to do your personal nighttime self-care routines. Perhaps your one micro-habit is to not do work at home after 6:00 p.m. or avoid TV past 9:00 p.m. Do you get the idea? In order for you to get to bed one minute earlier, you may need to change something up in your day or evening routine to help to make space to go to bed sooner than you do now. Maybe you won't need to. Maybe going to bed one minute earlier is so easy that you won't have to change anything. If that is the case, consider yourself lucky and go with it!

This is just the beginning. Be patient. You may be asking

yourself, "What difference is one minute going to have on my health?" Well maybe none. But we need to celebrate every rung on the ladder that gets us closer to our ultimate goal of a solid bedtime to get the amount of sleep we need to have our digestive systems and the rest of our body working at its best. That is a powerful reason. Our habits need to be powered by a strong *why*. It is our whypower that will sustain us, not willpower. Willpower runs out. Habits stick for a lifetime. If our habits hang around, we may as well make them so they assist us in reaching our goals. If you can master one tiny habit, you can master many. Even though you go to bed one little minute earlier, things have to take place for that to happen. Something has to change. Once you feel good about yourself for making that change and you start to feel better because of that change, trust me, you'll be eager for more. When I am following my own advice, I come upstairs between 10:00 and 10:30 p.m. Going upstairs signals the end of the day for me and I start my bedtime rituals...brushing my teeth, journaling, light stretching, meditation, and getting into my jammies. When I don't follow my own advice, I stay up later, watch too much TV, skip most of my evening self-care rituals, and usually wake up unrefreshed. All I have to do is come upstairs earlier...that's it. It's one tiny habit that sets off a mind- and body-improving ritual! I hope you implement your one tiny sleep-promoting habit and have pleasant dreams.

Chapter 18
Eating

Why Eating is Important

What about all those commercials for food? Tacos, ooey-gooey sweets, and baked goods. What gets you drooling? Pizza ads? Or the chocolatier making candy? We are certainly presented with many alluring and unhealthy choices every day whether you are watching ads on TV or simply walking through the breakroom at work. We are a culture that eats for pleasure with little regard to health. Allow me to be dramatic for a moment. Pause.

Nutrition is the be-all and end-all in your own personal health. Barring any super-dangerous habits such as smoking or drug addiction, your nutrition is a great place to start to improve your health. I tell my clients who want to take a pill or have a shot to lose weight, that **nutrition** is the secret weapon. Our bodies will release weight if they are getting the proper nutrients. Oftentimes, people want to fast, or eat only certain kinds of food to lose weight. I can write a whole book about how to lose weight without being obsessed with food or the scale, but let's turn our attention to the overall premise of the book, and that is to cure ourselves of digestive issues. Imagine if eating well could help reduce or eliminate our troubled digestive issues. Imagine if we didn't need all the medications to feel good. Imagine if just eating to suit your nutritional needs was all it took. Well, guess what? It can be. Read on to see what I mean.

Eating a healthy, balanced diet can have a lot of benefits for digestive issues. Food can be thy medicine. Just take a look at all the reasons why:

Reducing inflammation: Certain foods can trigger inflammation in the gut for certain people, leading to digestive issues like bloating, diarrhea, and abdominal pain, to name a few things. Eating foods rich in anti-inflammatory properties like fruits, vegetables, whole grains, and healthy fats can help reduce inflammation and improve digestive health.

Promoting healthy gut bacteria: The gut is home to trillions of bacteria that take part in digestion and overall health. Eating a diet rich in fiber, probiotics, and prebiotics can help promote a healthy balance of gut bacteria, which can improve digestion and reduce the risk of digestive issues.

Managing symptoms of digestive disorders: Certain digestive disorders like irritable bowel syndrome (IBS) and Crohn's disease can cause symptoms like abdominal pain, bloating, and diarrhea. Eating a diet that is low in trigger foods and high in nutrients can help manage these symptoms and improve quality of life. Be sure to discuss with your provider to let them know how you are working to improve your nutrition.

Supporting overall health: Digestive issues can be caused or exacerbated by other health conditions like obesity, diabetes, and heart disease. Eating well can help manage these conditions and improve overall health, which can in turn improve digestive health.

We can all agree that these things are important whether you have digestive issues or not! Now that we are armed with a big WHYpower, we can easily see why it's worth making the effort to eat better.

I will remind you again that it is important to speak with your doctor or a registered diet tian to develop a personalized plan that meets your specific needs. Your physician knows the specifics of your body and your medical history. Be sure to partner with them to make a plan that will help you reach your specific goals.

What Habits to Start With

Do you remember how I said it was a challenge for me to suggest what specific micro-habit to work on first for a better sleep routine? Well, it's even more of a challenge for me to suggest a starting point for you because there are so many parts to eating well, and there are so very many different health and digestive goals. If you want to start somewhere, you would want to know if you have any specific illnesses because there could be an eating protocol for that specific illness. Some folks reading this book may want a healthier eating lifestyle, and others may want to lose weight. That's one reason it's difficult to suggest which habit for you to work on first.

Once you've established the goal, the next part is to figure out what you already do well regarding nutrition in your day and what challenges you navigate. For example, I have a client who rarely ate during the day, and when she did, it was fast food, chips or cookies. Because she was so busy and felt as though she had no time to eat, we started with healthy packaged meal replacements. She was able to get some nutrition using healthy grab-and-go food with a structured meal plan that I use in my coaching practice. She was still able to stay as busy as she liked while we found an easy way to add nutrition to her day. A tiny tweak in her day led to her having more energy and feeling the difference between eating junk food vs. nutrient-dense food. If we just stopped right there, it would be enough to dramatically improve her health. If she wants to take more steps, she certainly can.

I have another client who has no interest in eating until nighttime, and then, not surprisingly, she overeats. So she is working on just adding protein powder to her morning coffee so she could get the feel of what fueling her body feels like. One client who has an inflamed digestive system needs to eat more foods that are anti-inflammatory, or less acidic. For him, we started with simply finding some plant-based recipes that were easy to make so he could always have food on hand to eat to build this new lifestyle.

Choosing the big goal, then picking one tiny habit to help you steadily get to your bigger goal is of utmost importance. This is a good place about which to consult with a coach, an accountability partner, or a healthcare provider. It's that important. Most people don't want to take it one micro-habit at a time. They want to go big. I don't discourage going big, as much as I want to promote sustainability. As long as you have the micro-habit in place, you can do more. If doing more doesn't work, remember to still consider it a win if only you accomplish the micro-habit, OK? That is very important.

Jim Rohn's quote says it all:

"Success is a few simple disciplines, practiced every day; while failure is simply a few errors in judgment, repeated every day."

— Jim Rohn

Smaller habits are easier to master, so it is easier to accumulate wins. When you accumulate wins, you build trust in yourself. Building trust in yourself is important in habit formation because we need positive talk to move forward and not sabotage our efforts. When you build wins and trust in yourself, you change your view of yourself to a person who can implement a new habit and become a person with a growing piece of this new identity. Then you can build and build toward the best version of yourself. Isn't that exciting? We can always move forward and accomplish new things, and be winning all the time. So let's not waste any time. Let's get to how we form a micro-habit to help us create better eating habits.

How to Form the Habits

We know that your macro-habit is to resolve your digestive issues and lead a vibrant life, leaving behind any worry that your digestive issues will flare up at the most inopportune time. Hopefully you have also chosen your micro-habit to start your focus on this lifestyle approach to healing. Assuming you have that, it is simply a matter of making sure it is small enough to easily accomplish. Some examples from my clients are things like: having fresh-squeezed lemon juice daily, eating one extra healthy snack each day, or adding one extra vegetable to their daily diet. One of my clients is a menopausal woman working to reduce the amount of sugar she eats, so her micro-habit is to simply record her daily grams of sugar. Her ultimate goal is to keep it below twenty-five grams of added sugars. She will eventually replace most added sugars with natural ones. As we begin to implement a new habit, we want it to be so small of a task and so specific that if it gets late in the day, you can still accomplish it. Remember we are working to build wins, confidence, and trust in ourselves.

Accountability is such an important topic that it will have its own chapter in this book. For now, allow me to bring it up briefly to say that eating routines are a simple way to be accountable. You could have an accountability eating partner. You could throw a stone and hit dozens of folks who are working on their health around nutritional and/or digestive issues. Find one and partner up. Call or text each other daily to tell each other what you have accomplished. Trust me: when you know you are going to be checking in daily with someone, it keeps your task top of mind.

Another fun accountability choice is tracking your behavior. Being an elementary-school teacher at heart, I find lots of fun ways to graph daily behavior goals. For folks who like to have a list and check things off, this is a good one. The graph becomes an accountability partner because you want it to be all filled out when you are finished with it.

Besides making the goal small and finding ways to be accountable to that goal, we need to talk about the structure of getting the task done in a habit-forming, permanent way. For example, my client who wanted to add lemon juice to her daily diet to ease her digestive woes made sure she drank it before she had breakfast. She left the lemon on the counter each night to give her a cue, or reminder. The goal was to have it before she started to prepare breakfast. For the accountability piece, it "counts" anytime of the day she has the lemon juice. We set up the pre-breakfast time because having breakfast was already a rock in her morning routine. When you can pair a new habit with one that strongly exists, it allows for more success. Remember this is called habit stacking: pairing a solid habit with one you are working to implement. It's efficient.

Of all tips on how you can implement eating habits to serve your goals, remember the main idea is to make **small**, incremental improvements. The ease with which you can incorporate these changes will lead to their permanence.

The last category of habits to develop is in the area of self-care. This is a fun topic because it can encompass so many things. Let's dig deeper into this popular, yet underutilized and sorely needed habit.

Chapter 19
Self Care

Why Self Care is Important

It's wonderful that self-care has become a popular topic. Thankfully, emotional well-being is now seen as a legitimate form of healthcare. Especially since the pandemic, more people recognize the benefits of tending to their emotional well-being. We talk about anxiety and depression a bit more freely now. Heck, there are even commercials and public-service announcements about such emotions. I am thrilled about that. Now, instead of shamefully sweeping those emotions under the carpet, we can feel normal for having them and actively look for solutions for working through them. Good companies even recognize the need to create a workplace environment where each employee is seen as an individual and given breaks because they now know that breaks in work lead to good mental health, which leads to more efficiency and productivity. Perhaps they have events or guest speakers to foster a community feel. It's exciting that this is becoming more mainstream in the workplace. Now that we know self-care is a legitimate practice to incorporate into our lives, let's delve a little bit into what happens when we put our own self-care and mental health on the back burner. I'll start this section with a client story to demonstrate how important self-care is to your physical health as well as your emotional health.

Sarah wanted to lose weight and reduce the stomach ailments she was experiencing, such as gas, bloating, and constipation. She was actually eating well and she was not sedentary. She was exercising a few days a week and was on her feet most of the day at work. You may be wondering what was holding her back from losing weight and settling her digestive issues. Well, it turned out that she had a very stressful home life raising two daughters as a single parent. She was an elementary school teacher, too. Anyone who has taught elementary school knows that there is a ton of stress in the classroom caring for so many individuals who need love and attention. Additionally, she had an administrator who did not support her.

Sarah worked hard to get all her healthy habits in place. After all, being the breadwinner in the family, she needed to be alive for a very long time to raise her girls. It was at this point we started to talk about what self-care was.

The definition of self-care is: the practice of taking action to preserve or improve one's own health. Anything you do to soothe yourself, comfort yourself, or move you closer to a deeper state of well-being can be considered self-care. With this definition in mind you can understand the importance of cultivating habits that provide a greater sense of well-being. This is what I got across to Sarah. She argued that she had no time to do laundry let alone something extra like self-care. I understood and asked her to come up with a list of things she liked to do but didn't have time for.

She reluctantly gave me a lengthy list.

My next question to her was to ask if she would just clear five minutes per day for self-care as a way to lessen stress, improve digestion, and maybe even lose weight. She said "yes," and from her list chose to dance for five minutes. She could do it alone. She could do it with her girls. She could do it in the morning, afternoon, or evening. All that mattered was that she danced for five minutes every day. Well, she started this new routine every morning. Her daughters were eager to join her, so they became extra cooperative in the mornings to get ready for school. All three of them looked forward to this part of the morning because it was fun. It added good energy, laughs, exercise, and good times. Imagine starting off each day with a dance party!

I'm guessing you already know what results she had with her physical issues or I wouldn't be writing about it, right? With the disclaimer that these results may not be typical for everyone, I will share with you that Sarah did start to lose weight and her digestive issues were nearly gone within a short amount of time. Seems too simple, right? I would agree except I have read the literature on how impactful reducing stress can be. If the body is a vessel that the mind feeds, we need to be thinking and feeling more positively. That is easier said than done when our lives have so much stress in them. However, when you see something as powerful as five minutes of dancing change the whole milieu of a family's morning routine and reducing a single mom's stress enough to help her release weight and dramatically ease her digestive issues, it's time to take a look at how we can incorporate self-care practices into our daily lives. What helps our mind helps our bodies. That's so powerful.

Self-care leads to a better-functioning immune system. Self-care also leads to energy improvement, stress reduction, better sleep, better concentration, and feeling happier. When you enhance your wellbeing, you are healthier. This is why I am mentioning it in this book on learning how to heal naturally. This is something that is good for our health and it feels good to do!! Read on to explore which self-care habits are best suited for you.

What Habits to Start With

Well, well, well. Where are we to start? Every single person is going to be different. What may soothe and calm me may be irritating to you. I suggest you start by making a list of things you enjoy, just like Sarah did. The list can have activities that are free, activities that only last a few minutes, and activities that can be done alone or with someone else. Think of something that you like to do but maybe feel like it's a luxury so you put it on the back burner. Now that you know some of the benefits of self-care, you are more likely to get to it each day. Here are some ideas, just to get your brain thinking about what could go on your list:

- A bath
- A facial
- An at-home beauty treatment
- A phone call to a friend
- Sit alone in the car before going home
- A walk

- Light a candle
- Chant
- Sing
- Have a cup of tea
- Do a puzzle
- Buy flowers
- Declutter an area in your home or office
- Get a massage
- Give yourself or get a manicure/pedicure
- Hug someone
- Listen to your favorite music
- Watch or listen to something inspirational
- Watch a sunset or sunrise
- Get out in the sunshine
- Go to a farmers' market
- Breathe deeply
- Take a nap
- Go to the library or bookstore
- Dance
- Do a social media detox

The examples above are just the start. The list can go on and on. Remember that self-care is a necessity, not a luxury. Start right now and make a list of five to ten go-to self-care activities you can readily do when you feel like you are falling apart and need some time to reset. Think about things that bring you joy. If your list is short right now, wait and see how it expands when you start to give it some thought.

How to Form the Habits

Now that you have your list of self-care desires, you need to figure out where it is going to fit in your daily routine—into an already busy, packed schedule. I would suggest squeezing it in daily. Remember not every self-care activity takes a lot of time. For example, if you are dancing, it could be to one song, or for five minutes. You decide. Figure out how you can get a short activity in daily. Maybe a day or two each week you can do something longer, like a mani/pedi or pilates.

The key to implementing this self-care habit is to schedule it and put it in the calendar. Treat it as an appointment and keep it.

Until you have these times solid in your schedule, I suggest using Sunday nights to decide where you can put your new activities on your calendar. I look to see what is on my calendar and figure out where I can add a self-care activity without adding any stress to my schedule. If I know I have back-to-back appointments, then perhaps that is a day to simply listen to an inspirational podcast as I am driving home. Or I may sit in the car for a few minutes before going to my next appointment. Think of a self-care activity that doesn't take much time. It should be something that relaxes you and brings you joy. Do not make this another dreaded task that needs to be accomplished daily. View it as joyful medicine to the soul and make it a sacred practice. In short, the secret to implementing this habit is to schedule it in your calendar and make sure to do it daily. Keep your list handy, too. You will most likely be thinking about self-care ideas more and new ideas will come to you. The key is to get them on your ever-growing list so you will have a huge list to draw on when you are scheduling activities. Once the self-care habit is securely in place, you may not even need to schedule it anymore; you will just be used to it being a part of your normal daily life. You will be a happier person now that you are prioritizing your well-being. This reduction of stress will act as an anti-inflammatory to your whole body, which will obviously have a positive effect on your digestive system as well.

Chapter 20

Accountability

Why Accountability is Important

In short, accountability is taking responsibility for one's own behaviors. Sounds simple, right? It can be. How you make yourself responsible for implementing your new behavior can also be simple, and you have a lot of choices. There are so many ways to incorporate accountability into your routine. I will describe some broad options. You can see which ones resonate with you. By the end of this section, you'll be able to create your own form of accountability that will be most effective for you.

What Habits to Start With

By now you are most likely motivated to implement all of the habits I've mentioned in this book. May I strongly suggest that you start with only one! Start with the one that is easiest so you can build some wins, gain confidence, and **feel** better. Once you have chosen the habit to start with, you will need to add a layer of accountability to ensure you are actually implementing your plan. Here are some specific types of accountability from which you can choose.

The first type of accountability is a **tracker**. A tracker is a fancy word for documenting your behavior. Let me give you some examples and you will totally understand.

1. **Calendar:** A calendar can be used to simply check off or cross out the day you accomplished the micro-habit you chose to work on.
2. **Charts:** These are so varied and can be straightforward or super creative. I have used charts that are block letters divided up by the days in a month. You just color in one day at a time. It's fun, colorful, and you can easily see what days you met your goal. Another type of chart is one where you add tally marks on the days you accomplish your task. It can also be more of a notebook where you write a narrative of the desired goal... what you did, what time of day, how you felt, and so on. Many of my clients opt to have a notebook where they write their daily wins. There are many different options on the internet that you can print out. It can be very simple or very elaborate and everything in between. Choose something you are most likely to do or you will not get the accountability results and implementing the new habit may become more of a challenge. Another reason why you want to pick an accountability tool that resonates with you is because it will **feel** good. Instead of focusing on what we do wrong, we focus on what we are doing right and that **feels** better. The positive

reinforcement also encourages us to do more, so we continue to see results feel good, and build trust in ourselves that we will do what we say we will do. We actually prove to ourselves that we are becoming the person we set out to be. Accountability is very powerful.

I remember when I was implementing the habit of meditation. My micro-habit was to take ten deep breaths in a day, and my macro-habit was to meditate for twenty minutes. If I did the ten deep breaths then I got to color in my tracker. Well, I missed a day. And I missed a couple of other days. I missed four days in all. I remember starting to berate myself for the four days I missed. Then, it dawned on me that I met my goal **twenty-six** days of the month! I was not perfect, but I did something twenty-six times in a month that I previously had wanted to but never done!! Big Win! My point in telling you this story of me implementing a new habit is to show you that the data you collect can be used to show what a rock star you really are. It's irrefutable evidence that you are working toward a goal. I was becoming a person who meditates! So many times, we can get a boot-camp mentality about change. In other words, it's all or nothing. No pain, no gain. I believe in the opposite. We need to learn how to create and implement a new behavior that will be sustainable. While I absolutely think it's a big deal to do this, it doesn't have to be brutal...which is how I view boot camps. That "boot camp"approach is just not a sustainable or enjoyable path to help me grow into my goals. If it is for you, go for it.

The second type of accountability is doing something in a **team, group, or community.** It has been said that you are a reflection of the five people you hang around most. If you are hanging around people who are not into improving their health, or worse, they have no health-promoting behavior, you are likely to fall prey to their unhealthy behaviors. When you want to break the chains of old behavior, you need to shake up who you hang out with. If your family are the people with the bad habits, most times we don't want to leave them, so we need to add people to support us. One such way is to find a group.

I will often create a **Facebook group** to accomplish this. It is amazing how many people are wanting to improve behavior to get their desired results. I guess it shouldn't really be surprising. We all need the support of others to move forward. It could be for encouragement, comradery, or tips. It's always easier to receive help from someone who has been or is going through the same thing as you. It's also fun to share your wins in these groups. I just finished a plant-based masterclass on Facebook. The group had replays, assignments, and a community waiting to share. The community became a place to get more information about new recipes or to ask questions. It was a place for encouragement, sharing wins, and feeling a sense of pride. My eating absolutely changed from the class, and the first place I wanted to share that win was in the group. We had a shared experience, so I knew they would appreciate what I was saying. This group absolutely helped to solidify my new education and my new habits. The group added a deeper level to my success.

Perhaps it's easier for you to get a **group together at work**. You could create a wellness challenge or organize walkers at lunch time. It will all depend on what you'd like to accomplish. Doing some sort of an activity together naturally creates accountability. You may not feel like walking at lunch time, for example, but if you have a group of people waiting for you, it's kinda hard not to go. Being part of a community lends itself to being lifted up and taking inspired action. These groups can be formed at work, in church, on social media, or just about anywhere. It only takes one person willing to create the group to get the ball rolling. Perhaps that person can be you!

The third type of accountability is a personal **accountability partner**. This could be a friend, spouse, work buddy, or family member. They do not even need to live in the same house. An accountability partner can offer support, call you out on your excuses, and share the journey with you. The two of you can decide the format that works best for each of you. You may decide things like:

- How often you are in contact
- If you will be writing things down, talking, texting, sending emails, or video conferencing
- If you will be journaling, or using some type of tracker

Once you get the routine established, you are off to the races getting your new routines in place. If you are a social person, this will be fun for you. You'll definitely be sharing quality time with your partner as you both work to establish habits to reach your goals.

And finally, while there are many more ways to create accountability, the last one I will mention is **coaching**. It will not come to a surprise to anyone reading this book that I am an advocate of coaching. Being one myself says it all, right? I hire coaches for myself, too. If you are always learning and growing, then you are always new to something that you'd like to be better at.

Having a professional coach to work with is beneficial because they can help with mindset, which is difficult to work on alone. Being objective, they can help to uncover blind spots and provide different perspectives that will hopefully make us grow and learn. They can provide structure, accountability, and support to move you toward your goals in a sustainable way.

Results are motivating, so the goal-attaining cycle continues!

Having someone to celebrate your wins with is my favorite part. Feeling lifted up is important for our mental and emotional health. Lifting each other up just isn't done enough in our lives. We tear others down and we tear ourselves down. I find that I am often teaching my clients how to celebrate their wins. Many times, they want to tell me about the "bad thing" they did this week instead of all the good choices they made that week. I like to flip the script on that.

I start all my coaching sessions by saying, "Tell me some of your wins for the week." This simple request helps them retrain their brain to find out what they are doing right all week long. They are thinking about or documenting their wins so that they can come to me prepared to share. This is how the mind transformation begins! A shift in their thinking from what they did wrong to what they are doing right is huge!

When I was an elementary school teacher, all I did for the first week of school was instill habits like pushing in the chairs, raising your hand to talk, and lots of other rules. My number-one tactic to get a classroom full of six year olds to cooperate was to praise, praise, praise them for everything I wanted them to do. "Good job sitting down, Johnny, "or "I like the way you raised your hand, Suzy," or "Oh my goodness, Timmy put his name on the top of his paper and I didn't even have to ask him to write it. Way to remember the rule, Timmy!"

I would say statements like those all day long. And guess what? I had well-behaved classes every year. They were pleasant-tempered and I rarely had to enforce rules during the year because they were just taught to do the correct things as part of the normal routine. They learned a new routine. A routine that would build them success in this new environment. My friends, this did not happen by luck. Each year I created a new, positive environment. How did I do that year after year? It's all about how I helped my students install habits joyfully. Making the process of learning a lot of new habits feel positive helps each of us lean into the change with more courage. It's not a place of consternation. It's a loving, understanding place where grace is given as often as needed. This safe, non-judgemental zone promotes activity that will promote good educational habits.

I shared my classroom experience as a roundabout way to say that being positive with ourselves is a skill. It can be developed. I believe this is an important piece to the coaching-style puzzle that is most successful. There are some coaches that will motivate around pain points and fear. That works for a lot of people. It doesn't work for me, which is why I am partial to a positive approach. I have had decades of success with this as an educator, with my clients, and in my personal life. Learn to praise yourself for the steps you take to improve yourself, or hire someone while you are learning to build that habit!!

Suffice it to say, working with a coach is a great way to efficiently implement new habits to help you reach your goals. Whether it is a tracker, a community, an accountability partner, or a coach, make a decision and then set out to put it in place. This is a way to make your goals visible. The more you are seen, the more you can accomplish.

How to Form the Habits

Whatever accountability tool you decide to implement, it's very important to take this activity seriously. It is a stepping stone to accomplishing your micro-habits and ultimately your bigger goals. It gives you information about what you are doing and where you are going. It's feedback to help you redirect your behavior if you are off track, or celebrate if you are on track and directly headed to your goals!

My suggestion is to start with a decision about which form of accountability will work best and get that set up first. Whether it is some form of trackers, a like-minded community, an accountability partner, or a coach, incorporate accountability somehow. I promise you it will make a huge difference in the success you have building your new habits. Make it a priority. If the idea of accountability seems like just another thing you are adding to your day, go for the easiest, least time-consuming tracker of them all. Put a checkmark on your calendar, or keep tally marks on a piece of paper. That will literally take seconds and it can be enough.

You may not need the accountability once the habit is built. It is a temporary piece of the habit-implementation puzzle that can lead to awareness and sustainability of your sought-after goal. I strongly suggest that you make it a priority in the goal-attaining process.

Chapter 21
Mindset

One of the most important messages in this book is that mindset matters. Why would I bring this up in a book about digestive issues and creating health in one's life? I will gladly tell you. There is a strong link between mindset and health. A positive mindset can boost your immune system. It can lower stress, which makes you less susceptible to illness and disease. Part of creating a positive, or growth mindset is to take a look at how we think. Our thoughts are constantly running their own script in the background of what we do all day, every day. We need to create awareness of them. In case our thoughts are not serving us well, we need to challenge them and flip the script.

Becoming more and more aware of the background dialogue that goes on constantly in our minds is key. We have the power to transform those thoughts. When we become the observers of our thoughts, we can challenge and redirect our thoughts. It takes some mental discipline after we've created this awareness. I'll go through a few examples of how you can work on mindset and awareness.

But first, let me share how this applies to my own journey. I would not be writing this book if I did not take control over my emotions. When I initially thought about it, I felt embarrassed. Here I am an expert in the field of health and I went ten years experiencing pain, bloat, and fear about what was actually wrong with me. I could have easily not written this book, avoided risking any judgment, and just taken my health win, and been on my merry way. My mindset helped me to realize that by writing this book, even if I only helped one person, it would all be worth it. It is the classic glass half full, or glass half empty. My mind tells me to be appreciative that I have the glass at all. I can be bound by fear and not share my personal journey, or I can open up about it and possibly help people.

Sharing Our Journey

Sharing your experience is one powerful way to process and digest the changes you've made and are still making, physically and emotionally. As a bonus, you can be an inspiration to others. I encourage my clients to share their health transformations for the same reasons I am sharing my story with you: to inspire. Sometimes when we are living our lives, crawling our way out of some physical or emotional hole, we tend to want to hide and not share our story. It can be embarrassing that we were in the hole in the first place. We all fall into holes. How we get out of them is not only of value to you, but it can be a roadmap for someone else who is not as far into the health-transforming journey as you are. Boldly share your story because it can inspire others. It's also a way to process and proclaim your own path. Own it and share it. Sharing your journey gives extra meaning and purpose to your transformation because it allows others a well-lit path to follow if they so choose. So shine your light!

Comparative Reality

We sometimes live in the inner world of comparative reality. Do you know what that is? It's when we judge where we are compared to someone else. Social media can exacerbate this when you see the highlight reel of other people's lives. Inevitably the folks posting have more friends, more fun, a better career, and a happier family than we do. We have all seen those celebratory posts and thought less of ourselves after viewing it. It's natural. I invite you to do two things when you find yourself in this comparative-reality mindset to get out of it as soon as possible.

Find Your Joy

First, evaluate your own personal joy. Perhaps you are already leading the dream life; it just may not be the standard look of the mainstream culture of success, money, and fame. The main population may be celebrating things you don't really want. Even if you do want what they have, maybe they have glorified their success by leaving out the parts about the grueling behaviors and the moments they missed out in other areas of their lives. Perhaps they have leaned heavily into the one goal they achieved but not acknowledging all the losses they accrued along the way. The fact of the matter is, we have no idea what happens in another person's life. There is no real way to tell. So many people are wrapped up in facades and images that they give us all a false sense of what success is and what it looks like. I suggest that you may very well have many successes building up, but you may not have noticed because the one goal, the one title, or the one rank you want eludes you. When you compare your life to the highlight reel of someone else's life, you may feel less successful. Start watching to see how often you do that. It is the first step to being able to put a stop to living in a comparative reality mindset.

Take record-breaking, professional tennis player, Novak Djokovic, for example. He is 34 years old (which is old in professional tennis years). Just today, as I am writing this chapter in my book, he made history and won his twenty-third Grand Slam victory. During the awards ceremony he thanked his opponent, the crowd, the tournament director, and so on. When he got to his coach he thanked him for putting up with him in the last few weeks as pressure was building. He took ownership of the hard work, the consistency and the ugly moments. Thankfully, he painted a more realistic view of what led to the celebration. It is but one moment in a long stream of moments that included eating right, scheduling tournaments sensibly, working out daily, and many other habits. It was a moment he has been cultivating for decades.

Imagine if I had a comparative-reality mindset and compared myself to Novak. I would be immobilized with personal doubt about the deficiencies in my own tennis game. Instead I feel inspired by him. His authenticity inspires me to emulate his processes...in other words, form habits that will move me closer to my tennis goals. It is about being consistent with the habits of success that eventually lead us down the path of success. We can then begin to evaluate our success not only by the results we get, but also by the habits we put in place. Goal attainment is on the other side of consistent, intentional behavior.

Celebrate Wins

After you evaluate your successes and your joys in your own meaningful way, I suggest that you celebrate the hell out of them consistently. Celebrating your wins daily is a sure-fire way to bring on more wins that will get you closer to that ultimate goal you've set for yourself. I assert that success is about increasing the enjoyment of the journey along the way to your goals as much as it is attaining the goal. Creating ways to foster this process-loving mindset is everything. Embracing the tedious tasks that we do repeatedly is what I call *process-oriented success*. In other words, we need to embrace the steps along the way and form them into habits, or we won't have the consistency needed to reach our goals. If we celebrate this process as we develop sustainable habits, we are sure to reach our goals. Learning to celebrate each small step and mini-accomplishment along the way will be the vehicle to actually take us the whole way. It's all about feeling grateful in the moment for what you are doing and who you are becoming.

It's probably obvious by now that my compelling desire is for people to get to process and realize their accomplishments. For most of our lives we downplay our light. We all do it at one point or another in our lives. When someone compliments you, you say, "Oh that was nothing." Or if they compliment your clothes, you quickly say "Thanks. It was so cheap, I got it on sale." Can you identify this type of downplay? We tend to minimize our wins with big and small things. Who knows why? Perhaps we all have an underlying feeling of inadequacy. A lot of people run around feeling as if they are not enough. Maybe they were told this by someone important growing up. Perhaps inadequacy came in school when they were not in the smart reading group, or even taking a Zumba class when they could not follow the steps.

When we celebrate wins, we can create more and more wins to celebrate. It's a retraining of the brain to focus on our accomplishments, not our disappointments. My goodness, we are humans. We are going to make repeated mistakes. Why do we tend to weigh those failures more heavily in our minds? It's a constant reminder of why we suck. Who wants those thoughts running around in our minds? Why would we want that voice to be guiding our thoughts? I want an encouraging voice in my mind, one who looks for the good in what I'm doing because that will train me to be kinder and more gentle with myself. It doesn't do me any good to have a harsh critic taking up space in my mind. You can train your brain to think of the positive in most situations. If we reprogram our brains to find our wins lots of things will begin to change. **We teach ourselves to create more of what we want!** (Read that again.)

Nowadays, I can very quickly turn anger at a person into a question that asks, "What is this telling me about myself?" Or I can be in traffic and I will view it as a positive because I usually give myself enough time to get somewhere, and I'm not in a rush. Chances are I'll be happy that I get to listen to more of my audiobook or a favorite song. Who knows? Maybe it's even the Universe preventing me from an accident that I would have been in if I was not stuck in the traffic. It's about cultivating a positive outlook. How can you turn your stressful or challenging experiences into a positive experience that benefits you? That's what I'll write about next.

Positivity

I could endlessly talk about positivity. I love this topic so much. It doesn't always come easily, though. It takes work to be positive. By work, I mean work in the mental gym with exercises such as the following: journaling, talking with a friend or therapist, writing in gratitude journals, or learning how to offer ourselves grace when we don't perform at our best. We need to create happiness rituals (or self-care rituals) that will bring us joy even when it gets challenging to do so. That's the work: creating and sustaining routines that we can get back to when we get derailed by life's challenges. We are all just doing the best we can to move forward. We all make mistakes as we learn. That's natural. We do not need to look at a mistake and form an opinion about who we are. We are not "less than" because we make mistakes. Learning something new yields mistakes and shows courage in trying something new. Does a toddler learn to walk on the first try? Not usually. Do we berate them for falling down? Or do we encourage them to try again and applaud them for all steps in the right direction? We need to treat ourselves like we would a toddler learning to walk. My goodness. The things we say to ourselves when we mess up would never be acceptable to say to a toddler. So let's not say those unkind words to ourselves, okay? My five-year-old granddaughter, Violet, once told me (when I didn't follow her coloring directions), "It's ok, Grandma. It's good to make mistakes!" She is so right. We celebrate the courage to try. We celebrate the consistency, not just the outcome.

When we get our mindset right, and build awareness to keep it right, working on our goals will be a more pleasant experience. Improving is a never-ending process for us as humans. We may as well experience joy along the way; not only does it feel better, but it also promotes well-being and that is ultimately what we are working towards. Imagine If we can solve, alleviate, or lessen our digestive issues with just a mindset shift. Wow.

Remember, this is not a quick-fix action plan. This is the lifelong journey of evolving into our best selves. When we get better, we may see another goal on the horizon. It's a love-filled journey and not a whip-cracking, whistle-blowing kind of deal. We simply celebrate reinforcing new structures and habits that serve us best.

Conclusion

You are your best line of defense to create a vibrant, healthy life.

What will your first step be to create the life you envision yourself having?

What I want for you is to heal fast and live long. I want you to be free of pain, and look for fun, new ways to promote health. It took me way too many years to finally figure out that I had a gallbladder issue. I was so discouraged from the medical delivery system that I tried many alternative practices, thinking I was healing, only to experience more pain and then having to go back to the drawing board and see what parallels I could detect. I wasn't wrong. I was thinking and researching and trying new things.

What I now know is that I could have done more, by finding a healthcare practitioner that I could partner with sooner. Someone who will not just write a prescription to solve the immediate symptom, but really work with me to find the origin of any issue. We need those partnerships. I encourage you to do all the research and try all the things. Equally, I encourage you to find the physician that checks all the boxes for you. Everyone has their own set of standards for who to choose and why. Sadly, with so many HMOs, we are at the mercy of the system that has the practitioners making quick guesses because they get reprimanded if they spend too much time with a patient. Can you believe that? It is still profit over people in corporate-run and insurance-based practices.

Why do you think we see so many concierge and direct-primary-care practices popping up? People want to go back to the olden days where your doctor knew the whole family. A doctor's visit was a family visit. I still remember Dr. Solomon from when I was pre-school age. He was a sage. Anything my mom needed to know medically, he was able to help her on the spot by answering a few questions for her. Nowadays, there are few neighborhood doctors that know all your family members. It is our responsibility to find the doctor who will become the quarterback on our health team. Find someone you trust and respect. If you have no medical issues, it's a great time to seek out a healthcare provider. If you have medical concerns it's an even better time.

Once you have a core physician, I encourage you to branch out. Acupuncture, chiropractic, healthy communities, and so many more can be part of your healthcare team. Without the energy healer I went to I wouldn't have stumbled upon my diagnosis. Explore. Learn. Experiment carefully with some reputable, alternative health practices.

Ultimately, **you** are in charge of your health. The information and data that only you can accumulate are invaluable, and they are the secret to unlocking the keys to your vibrant health. Please don't wait as long as I did to formulate a team that helps you get to the root cause of what's bothering your body. I recognize there are some ailments that are not curable. However, you want a medical team who won't simply react to your symptoms with no plan for a cure. In the meantime you can implement habits mentioned throughout this book to make you and your body the best that it can be. What will be your first step to create the health you envision yourself having?

Acknowledgments

To my closest girlfriends past and present: Randy, Erica, Debbie, Myriam, and Debra. I love you so much. You have encouraged me my whole life to just be myself. I am amazing and you women saw it first! You told me to always use my heart and my voice. You always saw me as beautiful...always and in all ways. I am beyond blessed to be surrounded with so much love. We share interests, time, thoughts, emotions, tears, laughs, and many great times. Thank you for really getting to know me and care about me. I feel more than ever that this is the key to a healthy, balanced life. I feel more loved in my life right now than I ever have been. You, my dearest friends, have cultivated that for me. I thank you eternally from the depths of my soul. I hope you see my positive wisdom in this book. I know with every fiber of my being that you are all incredibly proud of me. It is with all of you encouraging me that I can embrace my confidence and find a way to encourage and lift others in body, heart, and mind. I am immensely blessed and honored to have your friendship.

To Jessica, Christine, Tim, Jayk, Ruby and Violet, I love you all! It's because of you, I want to be my best.

Thank You

Reviews help authors grow their reach. If you gleaned wisdom from this book and find yourself mentioning it to friends and/or family, consider taking a moment to leave a review on Amazon amzn.to/3vjPfkO or **Goodreads.** Thank you for considering.

Your reviews help prospective readers decide if this is right for them & it is the greatest kindness you can offer the author.

About the Author

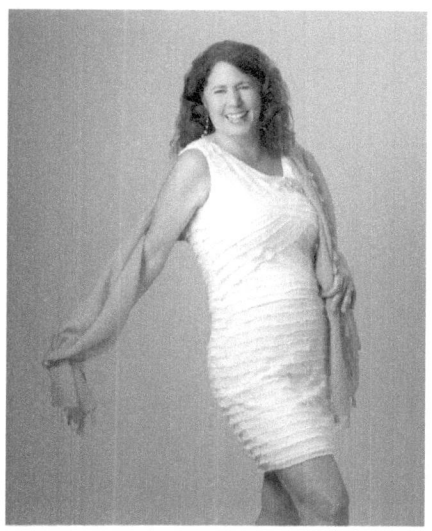

Sue's path changed dramatically when she experienced a physical transformation in 2009. She became passionate about paying the gift of health forward and went on to coach thousands of clients to improve their health.

This book was spawned from her ten-year quest to get answers about her own undiagnosed digestive challenges. Knowing she needed to stop her attacks of pain, seemingly associated with indigestion, she established lots of health-promoting behaviors and learned a lot about health and wellness. Now she is a health coach who wants to help people with digestive issues build a healthy lifestyle.

Sue coaches individuals, works with medical practices, and offers services in the corporate space. She does group presentations on many of the topics covered in this book.

To seek Coach Sue's services, go to her website: www.MyCoachSue.com

Book a complimentary discovery call.

Red Thread Publishing

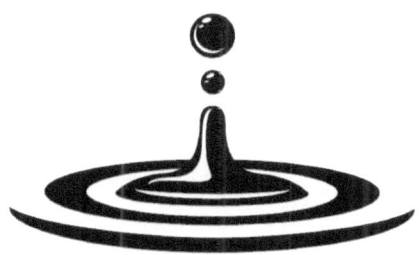

Red Thread Publishing is an all-female publishing company on a mission to support 10,000 folx to become successful published authorpreneurs & thought leaders.

To work with us or connect regarding any of our growing library of books email us at **info@redthreadbooks.com.**

To learn more about us visit our website **www.redthreadbooks.com.**

Follow us & join the community.

f facebook.com/redthreadpublishing

instagram.com/redthreadbooks

www.ingramcontent.com/pod-product-compliance
Lightning Source LLC
Chambersburg PA
CBHW020401130626
46549CB00006B/2380